TO
ALISON

THE BRAIN HAS A MIND OF ITS OWN

THE BRAIN

HAS A MIND

OF ITS OWN

INSIGHTS FROM A PRACTICING NEUROLOGIST

RICHARD RESTAK, M.D.

Crown Trade Paperbacks
New York

Published by Crown Publishers, Inc.
201 East 50th Street, New York, New York 10022. Member of the Crown Publishing Group.

Random House, Inc. New York, Toronto, London, Sydney, Auckland

Crown Trade Paperbacks and colophon are trademarks of Crown Publishers, Inc.

Manufactured in the United States of America

Library of Congress Cataloging-in-Publication Data

Restak, Richard M.

       The brain has a mind of its own: insights from a practicing neurologist / Richard Restak. — 1st ed.

              p.   cm.

Includes bibliographical references and index.

1. Brain—Popular works. I. Title.

QP376.R464   1991

612.8'2—dc20   91-12503

                                                              CIP

ISBN 0-517-88080-6

10 9 8 7 6 5 4 3 2 1

First Paperback Edition

CONTENTS

Contents

ACKNOWLEDGMENTS

Among the people who have contributed to this book, I am especially grateful to B. D. Colen of *Newsday*, who invited me to contribute essays to the "Discovery" section that he edits; Curt Suplee of the *Washington Post*, who provided advice and suggestions concerning what was worth writing about; Jerry Gross, who taught me the value of compression; Peter Guzzardi, who first suggested this project and provided invaluable help in seeing it to completion; and finally, Carolyn Restak, for her patience and understanding.

THE BRAIN HAS A MIND OF ITS OWN

o

INTRODUCTION

Take up writing. You have a talent for it," my mother encouraged me as long ago as I can remember. "Take up medicine," said my father. "As a doctor you can do something helpful for people every day of your life."

Because my childhood predated the rebellious 1960s I, very unrebelliously, decided to please both my parents. And I have been twice rewarded: both parents turned out to be right. Writing has brought me immeasurable pleasure and personal rewards, including the opportunity to see my thoughts transformed into the seven books I've written so far. Medicine has given me insights into the human heart that have informed and enriched my writing. In emergency rooms, clinics, and my own offices I've encountered pity, remorse, hatred, tenderness, and longing in their most dramatic forms.

Such intense glimpses into hearts and minds can be disorienting and numbing. You can't encounter raw emotion on a daily basis for years without having something dreadful happen. Some doctors take to drink, the comfort of readily available drugs, the pursuit of other men's wives, suicidal hobbies. Fortunately, I've largely avoided these paths to self-destruction by writing things down in an attempt to create order out of life's chaos and overstimulation.

1

Another benefit of being a doctor who writes is the balance demanded by these two very different activities. On those occasions when I literally can't sit still, I love the frenetic pace of a busy clinic. At such times I couldn't write a single sentence, much less an essay. The rhythm just isn't right. Only after the hyperactivity passes am I ready to write. The energy demanded then is purely psychic. I must combine receptivity—a passive process—with active inner exploration.

These cycles of activity and productive passivity aren't always mutually exclusive. There are times in the clinic or the office when I encounter a patient or a situation that I know I'll write about someday, and those stories often seem to write themselves. At other times the process is pure torture. When nothing is forthcoming, the doctor in me frets that I'm wasting valuable time, forgetting that before creation there must be germination.

What unites these two very different professions? As far back as I can recall I've been curious about why people do the unpredictable, amazing, and sometimes just plain crazy things that they do. What are the forces that motivate the con man, the serial killer, and the saint? How can emotions and moods be explained, controlled, perhaps even predicted?

I soon found out that only a limited number of professions offer the opportunity to explore such interests. Novelists, for example, are constantly concerned with the motivation and personality of their characters. The career of a novelist once appealed to me, but I felt then, as I still do today, that to spend one's life in the company of creatures of one's own making could get a little dicey.

What I sought was a profession that would enable me to indulge my interests in and curiosity about human behavior, and at the same time reduce some of the suffering in the world. It should therefore not surprise you to learn that I found psychiatry very appealing. But one formidable obstacle loomed in my path: my father.

A physician himself and eager for me to take up medicine as a career, he nevertheless was deeply hostile toward psychiatrists and psychiatry. On innumerable occasions he told me that psychiatrists didn't understand the bases for the illnesses they treat (an objection that to a large extent remains legitimate to this day). He was also convinced that many of those attracted to the specialty are themselves emotionally disturbed, and that their mental imbalance is often the motivating factor for selecting psychiatry as a specialty. As if those objections weren't sufficient, he added that my talents would be thoroughly wasted if I persisted in my plans to become a psychiatrist.

With that as an introduction to psychiatry, I entered medical school determined in this instance to defy his wishes and become a psychiatrist.

Early in training I realized that, exaggerated and one-sided though it had been, much of what my father had told me was true. At that time, the late sixties, very little was known about the causes of the major mental illnesses. In place of knowledge I encountered dogmatism and internecine conflicts. Freudians fought with Sullivanians, who battled the followers of Melanie Klein or Karen Horney.

A second surprise was finding out that psychiatrists at that time had little interest in the brain. With the exception of those few who were also neurologists (like Freud), they rarely stopped to consider if a particular mental or emotional illness could be the result of brain disease. But far more was involved here than simply a lack of interest in the brain. Many of the psychiatrists I came into contact with in the sixties and seventies were hostile toward those who suggested that the study of the brain might have something to offer. After several tangles during my psychiatry residency with psychiatrists of that persuasion, I shifted my interests and specialty training into neurology: the study of the brain and its disorders.

The last twenty years have witnessed dramatic new insights into the relationship of the mind and the brain. Thanks to the development of powerful tranquilizer and antidepressant medications, new techniques for imaging the human brain, and genetic studies showing that many emotional illnesses are hereditary and associated with physical alterations in the genome, the schism between psychiatry and neurology has narrowed. New to this more collaborative scene are hybrid specialists like myself, neuropsychiatrists, who bear testimony to the premise all behavior has its origin in the human brain and can be understood only in reference to the brain and its function.

Having chosen my first profession, I followed my mother's suggestion that I take up writing and thus began another. My first efforts, while I was still a neurology resident, consisted of opinion essays for the *Washington Post* on such subjects as euthanasia, psychosurgery, and genetic engineering. I also wrote some strictly reportorial pieces in the late seventies as a "stringer" for the *New York Times*. These included reports and comments on brainwashing, hypnotism in the courtroom, and biological psychiatry. After honing my writing skills, I began the first of the seven books on brain and behavior that I've written since 1975. Writing them made me change the way in which I looked at the world. And that change led directly to the book that you are about to read.

Understanding the brain provided me a deeper understanding of everyday life events. I found myself fascinated by the gait of someone walking in front of me, a momentary lapse of memory, or the execution of a perfect tennis return. The process was like putting on a pair of tinted sunglasses and finding from that moment on that everything in the world took on a special hue. Even something as ordinary as trying to ride a bicycle for the first time in many years underscored for me how the brain never forgets anything it has once learned—even though we may not be capable of putting that knowledge into words or even consciously recalling it. It inspired the essay in this collection "Thinking About Knowing." While taking a lesson in t'ai chi, that ancient Oriental exercise that is at once dance and martial art, I began thinking of the importance of form and the limits it places on the brain and its owner ("A Proper Form for Everything"). And speaking of ownership, do we "possess" a brain in the same way that we possess a kidney or a liver? Or is it more accurate to identify our brain with the essence of ourselves? In other words, is the relationship of a brain to a person that of an owner to a possession? Or should the relationship be more properly thought of as an identifying one: Are we our brains? This haunting philosophical question stimulated several essays in this book, including "Mapping the Spaces a Mind Can Enter" and "The Two Realities of the Mind."

Other essays of a more practical nature include something I first wrote for the *Washington Post*, "The Fiction of the Reasonable Man," which challenges the facile assumption that we are always capable, at least in theory, of acting unemotionally. As a result of what we have learned about the human brain we now know that such beliefs are simply wrong. Our brains are not organized the way judges and juries might wish. Any one of us, if we are sufficiently frightened or terrorized, can respond with extreme violence, no matter how "reasonable" we may consider ourselves. In addition, this inborn brain-based propensity for violence makes us particularly vulnerable to the effects of vividly portrayed depictions of violence in the movies and on television. So far this insight has been overshadowed and obscured by claims that television and movie violence is strictly a freedom of speech issue. In "Violence as News" I suggest that the issue reaches beyond civil liberties. It involves no less than our collective mental health. In "Those Eyes" and "Our Own Worlds" and "Anguish and Self-Destruction," I explore the fascinating emotional and ethical issues raised by patients suffering from irreversible brain damage, narcissism, and the impulse toward suicide. On some occasions the challenges I face aren't exciting or exacting. At those times the neuropsychiatrist can be most helpful by setting aside his or her own agenda for the patient and simply doing what is often the hardest thing of all: simply listening. "A Temporary Reprieve" and "The Listener" tell the stories of two such encounters. "Lucid Dreaming on Demand" and other essays treat the importance of dreams and how we can use them to learn more about ourselves. "When Ignorance Is Bliss" explores a situation faced by many doctors, patients, and relatives: When new tests predict that someone in perfect health will come down with an incurable, often fatal disease, should that person be told now? Or, as the essay suggests, are there times when it may be better not to know one's fate?

In the final essay, a response to the bill signed by President Bush declaring the 1990s the Decade of the Brain, I attempt to predict some of the future spaces the mind and brain sciences may enter during this last decade of the twentieth century. Much of this material developed as a result of my good fortune to serve throughout 1989–1991 on a congressional advisory panel called New Developments in Neuroscience. Our committee, composed of some of the leading neuroscientists in the country, evaluated where we stand in terms of understanding the brain and what we expect will be important over the next decade or so. Fascinating and, I'm sure, humbling surprises may lie in store for us. So far no person or committee has ever been able to foretell new developments in the neurosciences. Will a blue-ribbon congressional committee do any better? Stay tuned to find out.

In writing these essays and including them in this book, I've relied on two guiding principles. First, the subject should be relevant to the everyday life of my intended reader: a curious and intelligent person without formal training in or knowledge about the brain. Second, the essay should make the ordinary fresh and provocative.

Having read this far about who I am and how this book came to be, you may wonder: So what *are* you, finally, a doctor or a writer?

That same question was once put to Chekhov, one of my heroes. His answer was one I could never hope to improve upon:

"Medicine is my lawful wedded wife, writing is my mistress. When I tire of one, I spend the night with the other."

I hope that you will enjoy your next few nights with this book, *The Brain Has a Mind of Its Own.*

o

MY BRAIN AND I
ARE ONE

I once attended the wedding of a thirty-five-year-old patient who five years earlier had come to me after seeing in broad daylight the ghost of her dead first husband.

At our first meeting she told me about the ghostly visitor, but only after I had asked a simple question: "Has anything strange . . . you know . . . out of the ordinary ever happened to you?"

"Like what?" she responded, fixing upon me a pair of now fully dilated eyes.

She then revealed that on occasion she experienced a wave of fear accompanied by "strange sensations," such as a metallic taste in her mouth or a smell in the environment like that of burning rubber. On other occasions while in her home she felt as if everything had been "somehow altered." Sometimes the alteration involved her own sense of herself as somehow split into two people: an observer who commented on her actions, and an actor who carried them out. ("Yet both of them are me," she said.)

When I asked for further details, she said: "It's as if I'm a character in a science fiction novel who inhabits one dimension of reality while the rest of the world lives in another."

The electroencephalogram, which measures the brain's electrical activity, provided me with proof of what I already suspected. Karen's disturbed sense of herself originated from an epileptic discharge deep within the left temporal lobe of her brain.

The temporal lobe is responsible for our sense of connectedness, our personal identity, the feeling of belonging we get from familiar surroundings. When it functions normally, we have no apprehensions about who we are, our situation, or the nature of things. But when the temporal lobe is diseased, strange things can occur. A seizure originating in the temporal lobe can produce disorientation, feelings of having previously experienced events happening at the moment (déjà vu), or equally troubling feelings that familiar objects and people are new and vaguely threatening (*jamais vu*).

Another temporal lobe epileptic I once treated spent long hours in the middle of the night writing philosophy. He filled notebook after notebook with philosophical ramblings that in broad daylight he was able to recognize as not likely to be of much interest to anybody but himself. A serious man, he made me think of prophets and seers. At times his ruminations on the nature of the spiritual world became ecstatic, almost sexual. Dostoevsky, a temporal lobe epileptic, described the process in *The Idiot:*

There was always one instant just before the epileptic fit . . . when suddenly in the midst of sadness, spiritual darkness and oppression, his brain seemed momentarily to catch fire, and in an extraordinary rush, all his vital forces were at their highest tension. The sense of life, the consciousness of self, were multiplied almost ten times at these moments which lasted no longer than a flash of lightning. His mind and his heart were flooded with extraordinary light; all his uneasiness, all his doubts, all his anxieties were relieved at once; they were all resolved into a lofty calm, full of serene, harmonious joy and hope, full of reason and ultimate meaning. But these moments, these flashes, were only a premonition of that final second (it was never more than a second) with which the fit began. That second was, of course, unendurable. Thinking of that moment later, when he was well again, he often said to himself that all these gleams and flashes of supreme sensation and consciousness of self, and, therefore, also of the highest form of being, were nothing but disease, the violation of the normal state; and if so, it was not at all the highest form of being,

*but on the contrary must be reckoned the lowest. Yet he came at last
to an extremely paradoxical conclusion. "What if it is disease?" he
decided at last. "What does it matter that it is an abnormal intensity,
if the result, if the instant of sensation, remembered and analyzed
afterwards in health, turns out to be the acme of harmony and
beauty, and gives a feeling, unknown and undivined till then, of
completeness, of proportion, of reconciliation, and of startled prayer-
ful merging with the highest synthesis of life?"*

An encounter with a person suffering from temporal lobe epilepsy raises a question philosophers have argued about for centuries: What is the relationship of mind to brain? How can a
disturbance within a fairly circumscribed area of the brain produce
such transcendental experiences? Most experts have taken refuge
from such questions in a vague and untidy dualism that, until fairly
recently, was supported by our experiences with physics and machines.

Dualism, the metaphysical conception that body is separated
from mind, originated with the seventeenth-century philosopher
René Descartes. Descartes proposed that the body, especially the
brain, is a machine with functions that can be explained by the
mathematical laws of physics. But over the past sixty years physics
has changed greatly. According to the principles of quantum physics the observer cannot be meaningfully separated from the experiment that he or she is conducting. Indeed, the viewpoint of the
observer often determines what is recorded by the experiment.

The most famous example of the observer effect occurs in the
double-slit experiment, wherein a stream of particles is directed
toward a screen. A second screen, containing two long parallel
slits, is then placed between the stream source and the original
screen. With the two slits open the particles arrange themselves in
bands alternating with blank spaces in between. But when only one
slit is open, the particles fill in the blank spaces. "Particles or
waves? Which is the true picture?" asks physicist Fred Alan Wolf.
"It depends on which part of the experiment is being performed.

With one slit open, the stream is composed of particles. With two slits, it is composed of waves." The nature of what is being measured depends on how the observer sets up the experiment.

The observer effect holds true for brain/mind dualism, as well. When I listen to my patients tell me about a frightening vision or hallucination—something far removed from everyday experience— I'm encountering the world of mind. But if I record my patient's brain waves during a hallucination and detect an epileptic seizure within the temporal lobe, I've shifted my focus, like the scientist in the double-slit experiment, from one aspect of reality to another.

Marcus Raichle, head of the brain study group at the Washington University School of Medicine in St. Louis, suggests another way of thinking about such a paradox: "Because the brain is a physical structure, it exists in space; but the mind operates in time alone."

The brain as I stare at it depicted on a CAT scan or set out upon an autopsy table is very much an object. It takes up space; I can see it or its representation; I can pick up the autopsy specimen. We're talking about spatial matters here.

Mind, in contrast, can be captured only in the temporal dimension. My thoughts require time before I can communicate them to you in the form of words. Without motion or some form of behavior, mind cannot be inferred. Indeed, if I don't move or speak, can you really be sure I'm thinking at all?

The closer we look, the more difficult it is to maintain any neat division between mind and brain. Suppose I shout the word *fire* in a crowded theater. That word, *fire*, is conveyed by means of sound waves that stimulate the tympanic membranes in the ears of the listeners. Within milliseconds electrochemical events occur in the auditory nerve. They then traverse the labyrinthine pathway within the brain from auditory cortex to auditory association area to limbic system. There the word *fire* is loaded with fears traceable to the first caveman who burned his fingers before a campfire. Sound waves stimulate tympanic membranes, and physical alterations take place in the brain. Milliseconds later, thanks to the limbic involvement, the hypothalamus and sympathetic nervous system are drawn into the fray: heart rate increases, blood pressure rises, breathing becomes constricted and labored. The result: hundreds of people jump up from their seats to rush toward the exit—all in response to a concept conveyed by a mere word. Shouting the word *fire* exerted a powerful influence on matter. At a minimum the physical structure of the brain has been changed, albeit momentarily.

Other words and phrases of a different sort (*You're a failure; I want a divorce; I love you*) exert more permanent modifications within the brain. The PET scan of a schizophrenic or a manic-depressive shows a distinct variation from what, for lack of a better term, we call a normal brain. On the whole it's likely that these distinctions represent differences in the organization and function of the brains of those unfortunates who suffer from these illnesses. Alter the brain and you alter thoughts, feelings, and personal identity. And if you change an attitude or modify your own or someone else's behavior, you've worked a miracle, performed a successful experiment in psychokinesis: you've used the intangible mind to transform something in the physical world.

Mind can affect brain; brain can affect mind. But can either be separated from the other? Not any more than the other side of this paper can be separated from the side that you are now reading.

My experience with temporal lobe epileptics has raised a haunting personal question: How many of my own habits and propensities are determined for me by my brain? To what extent am I anything other than my brain? Is there any way of separating the brain from the person who just asked that question? My way of coping has been to fashion a simple mantra I repeat silently from time to time: "My brain and I are one. My brain and I are one." But even as I think and speak these words—my brain changing all the while as I do so—I still find it difficult to believe that this three-pound mass of protoplasm with the consistency of an overripe avocado is the seat of who I am, of who we all are.

o

MAPPING
THE SPACES
A MIND CAN ENTER

The geography of inner space permeates our language. "Where's your head at?" says one teenager to another. If somebody is daydreaming, we say, "Come down to earth. . . . Get your head out of the clouds." And "Do you know where I'm coming from?" is a question asked by many of us every day.

Such comments imply that the mind can dwell in several "spaces." But how does one identify which space anyone may be inhabiting at the moment?

You can understand the difficulty of that task by tracking your thoughts as they waft from one space to another. For instance, at the moment I'm sitting on my porch in Martha's Vineyard. I hear a bird outside the window behind me . . . and . . . this gets me thinking of a parrot that I'm considering buying . . . which stirs up memories of an Irish superstition told to me by my mother that parrots are unlucky. So far my luck in life has been pretty good, I reassure myself. Should I risk changing it? But I don't want to give in to superstitions.

Notice that all of the above thoughts were stimulated by my suddenly and briefly becoming aware of a bird. In a few seconds my mind had wandered from writing the essay that you are now reading to other spaces: desire for a parrot, anxiety about bad luck, cynicism regarding superstition.

At other times the mind wanders from one space to another in response to internal processes. A dream may awaken the sleeper and set off a chain of thought totally foreign to the concerns of waking consciousness. Acknowledging that the mind can exist in many spaces permits people to learn much about themselves.

Wandering from one space to another, the mind reveals a tapestry of thoughts and inner experiences that would remain hidden were we to tether the mind on too short a leash. "The following of thematic designs through one's life should be, I think, the purpose of autobiography," wrote Vladimir Nabokov in *Speak, Memory*. Do these thematic designs consist of anything more important than recurring thoughts and emotions that occupy consciousness, sometimes for extremely fleeting moments?

A topography of inner space would seem, therefore, to be extremely useful. But how can we construct such a map? I recently asked psychologist John Crook about this, and he suggested the following state-space continuum:

INTENTION

INTENSION + EXTENSION

ATTENTION

This grid, although extremely simple in construction, is very useful in defining mental space. For instance, most of the time our mind is involved in intending something (getting, changing, altering, etc.) about the external world (intention-extension). Maybe we want to change a job, get paid more, remodel a house. However, if we want to change ourselves—perhaps become more tolerant, eat less, give up smoking—the intending is similar, but this time is turned inward (intention-intension). Most of us, most of the time, are involved in the intention-extension space: we want to change something about the world. On infrequent occasions, on vacations or away from the office, we recognize that perhaps it's our inner attitudes that demand change (the intention-intension space).

At the other end of the vertical axis is attention: encountering the inner *and* outer world *without* trying to influence or change it in any way. A Zen monk sitting for hours looking out over the monastery garden is dwelling in this attention-extension space. A person attending to his interior *mental* processes without trying to alter them in any way is in the attention-intension space. This is a trance state induced through hypnosis or other means.

Cultures as well as personal style deeply influence which space you inhabit. For instance, most of us are part of what Crook refers to as the Western mind-set. In my own case, if I were less driven toward accomplishment, the sound of the bird mentioned a moment ago might have led me into the attention-extension space. Instead, my thoughts about whether I was going to acquire (intend to buy) a parrot drove me into the intention-extension space.

From personal experience, as well as professional, I've learned the value of letting my mind wander freely from one point to another on this state-space continuum. When you are overwhelmed with the desire for something that seems unobtainable at the moment (intention-extension), your energy can be renewed if you focus your mind with rapt attention on something—e.g., the play of sunlight on carpet or the sound of rain in your immediate surroundings (attention-extension).

To be complete and whole, we must have the courage to let our minds wander into every available space. We all live and travel on the same planet, but we are truly free only if we permit ourselves to visit at any time the different, exciting, and challenging worlds that exist solely within our own minds.

THE COMPASSIONATE BRAIN

S ome wit once said that people should be divided into two groups: those who believe that people can be so divided and those who don't.

A more useful division would be those who believe the world is stable—that seeing is believing—and those for whom the world consists of dynamic processes.

For the longest time, the human brain was included among those things that seemed to change very little over a lifetime. But this concept came to be doubted when neuroscientists learned that brain cells die off at a rate varying between fifty thousand and one hundred thousand per day. And at the level of synaptic connections between nerve cells, the attrition rate is even more incredible: we lose ten thousand synapses per second, according to Yale neuroanatomist Pasko Rakic. Yet despite these stupendous losses, most of us feel that on the whole we're smarter in our thirties and forties and fifties than we were during childhood, when our brain contained so many more neurons.

When I say "smarter," I'm not speaking here about IQ or the ability to pass a standardized test; indeed, most of us, if we took our college entrance test now, would perform *less* ably. No, by "smarter" I mean knowing more about how the world "works," how we can best achieve our ends, and understanding the events and interpersonal processes going on around us.

But how could a physical organ like the brain perform better with *fewer* cells? Such a conception contradicts everyday experience. Imagine a car or a television set, or any technical device for that matter, that would run *more* efficiently after the *removal* of many of its parts. Not exactly what you expect from a machine, is it?

And established concepts die slowly. The idea of the brain as a machine is firmly entrenched in our vocabulary. "He had a mental crack-up," we explain when one of our friends suffers an emotional illness. The same machine metaphor applies when we speak of our own mind as being "rusty," or unable to "grind out" solutions to certain problems. On other occasions our mind is "sharp as a razor" or "really revved up"; the "wheels are turning" within our heads.

Even when we don't speak of a machine, we tend to describe the mental processes mediated by our brain as immutable *things*. For instance, certain commonly employed phrases depict the brain as a delicate object that may be easily broken at any time. "Be careful what you say to him. His ego is easily bruised," describes a friend beset by insecurities and oversensitivities. "After the LSD experience his mind was simply shattered," or "She went to pieces when she was told of her child's death in the fire," or "His mind just snapped from the shock of it all." Granted that I'm mixing references to brain and mind fairly loosely here. Nonetheless, the overall flavor of the words and phrases used to describe mind, as well as brain, suggests an object, a thing, a substance.

Not everyone has always subscribed to the view that the brain, once it reaches maturity, changes very little thereafter. In 1874 Charles Darwin noted that domesticated rabbits had smaller brains than rabbits living in the wild. He suggested this might be explained on the basis of the close confinement experienced by domesticated rabbits during many generations. Sheltered from the threats to life in the wild, domesticated rabbits had less need for intellect, vigilance, and rapid responsiveness to threats from predators. In a sense, domestication had brought about in the rabbits a form of disuse atrophy in the mental sphere, similar to the atrophy of inactive muscles, joints, and ligaments. "Use it or lose it," as generations of physical education instructors have advised their students.

The idea that mental exercise can favorably modify the structure of the brain just as physical exercise can change one's bodily proportions is fairly recent.

In the 1920s Robert Tryon, a psychologist at Berkeley, observed that some rats ran mazes better than others. By inbreeding, he succeeded in establishing two strains, one maze-bright and one maze-dull. Over the next thirty years these strains were maintained separately from each other. In the 1950s two Berkeley scientists, a psychologist, David Krech, and a chemist, Melvin Calvin, set about investigating whether or not the brains of the two strains of rats differed in any way. They assumed that the bright rats would have more of a specific neurotransmitter, acetylcholine, in order to facilitate transmission across synapses. But because acetylcholine is very unstable and difficult to measure, the scientists concentrated instead on measuring the enzyme acetylcholinesterase, which breaks acetylcholine down into its components. A series of experiments proved the hypothesis correct: there *is* more acetylcholinesterase, and therefore more acetylcholine, in the brains of the maze-bright animals than in the maze-dull group. The rats' learning to successfully negotiate a maze had modified their brains' physical structure.

Although Krech, Calvin, and their associates were the first to test whether or not the brain could be modified by experience, they were not the first to suggest the possibility. Forty years earlier Nobel Prize–winning physiologist Ramón y Cajal had suggested that "cerebral exercise" could increase and enhance the connections between neural cells. Over the past thirty years Marian Diamond, professor of anatomy at the University of California at Berkeley, has continued this tradition of studying the influence of the environment on the structure of the brain. In *Enriching Heredity: The Impact of the Environment on the Anatomy of the Brain*, published in 1988, Diamond describes her findings. Overall, they deal a death blow to the idea of the immutable brain.

"Perhaps the single most valuable piece of information learned from all our studies is that structural differences can be detected in the cerebral cortices of animals exposed at any age to different levels of stimulation in the environment," she writes.

Diamond speaks of an "enriched environment," by which she means several animals housed together in a large cage with a variety of novel objects to explore and play with. An impoverished environment consists of rats in small cages containing neither objects nor companions. At its most basic, the enriched environment provides stimulation to the senses. In addition, such an environment provides novelty, new experiences, and, most important of all, information.

Although no one has ever come up with a totally satisfactory definition of information, I like best Jeremy Campbell's. "Change is the essence of information," he writes in *Grammatical Man: Information, Entropy, Language, and Life.* "A message source must be free to vary its messages, to send different sequences of symbols. There is no point in sending the same sequence over and over again." No point, indeed.

Environmental enrichment—more toys, more room to move around in, more companions, or just better nutrition—increases the amount of information delivered to the brain. New information leads to curiosity about other things, which, in turn, produces even more information. Most gratifying of all, this enrichment-enhanced brain correlation continues into old age and beyond. "The experimental environment is a major factor in maintaining the healthy older brain," says Diamond, who is convinced of the "potential of the cortical cells to respond to the information coming in from the environment."

Environmental influences on the human brain's structure and function take on a special significance in view of the fact that our environments are not only external, but internal as well. "All that we are is a result of what we have thought," says the unknown author of that ancient Eastern book of wisdom the *Dhammapada*.

But what effects on the human brain's structure and functioning result from the thoughts and emotions generated by the coercive and violent environments in which so many of us find ourselves?

Harvard psychologist Jerome Kagan observes:

> *The majority of Americans live and work in large metropolitan areas, far from family and childhood friends, and in frequent encounter with strangers who they suspect will exploit or frustrate them. These strangers will block access at crowded highway intersections, push ahead in long queues, and some may even cheat them when their roof leaks or when they elect surgery for a possibly infected gall bladder. It seems necessary that each of us be continually ready to resist exploitation and to display anger if threatened or forced to defend our property or dignity. Each person must have quick and easy access to the biological emotion of anger.*

Access to anger, coupled with its frequent expression, facilitates neuronal pathways within the brain subserving negative emotions. As a corollary to this, anger, hostility, and rage are more "natural" and expressible in the average city environment than, say, compassion. This is one of the reasons I've never really enjoyed living in large metropolitan cities. One must continually guard against the effect of such an environment: the blunting of one's sensibilities; the giving in to cynicism, anger, and frustration. Once established, conditioned reflexes of impatience, competitiveness, and petty resentments take their psychological tolls. Naturally, not everyone living in large metropolitan areas gives in to such emotions. But does anyone seriously suggest that there's nothing to be concerned about when one is constantly exposed to situations that engender such emotions? To turn the question around: Is there any evidence that a compassionate, loving, gentle environment can exert a beneficial effect on the brain?

"As we learned from our studies on aging rats, by giving our old rats a little tender loving care, we were able to increase their life span. Those rats that received additional attention lived longer than those who did not," writes Marian Diamond.

Within the brain tender loving care involves two-way communications between the cortex and the limbic system. Information is not just a matter of facts, symbols, and mental challenges, but includes care, attention, and other expressions of emotional involvement.

Personally I find Marian Diamond's findings both gratifyingly encouraging and morally challenging. If the brain is continually modifiable and enhanced by an enriched environment, then don't we all have a special responsibility to provide some enrichment to the environments of those around us? And if so, does this obligation extend only to our loved ones? Or does it also include our neighbors? Should it include our fellow citizens? We are confronting, in a different, more scientific guise, an issue that saints, philosophers, and sages have always held as one of our most important life decisions: What are the obligations of each of us for the well-being of all others?

Think about those obligations the next time you see an obviously mentally ill person coming toward you on the street.

Or when you see the outstretched, importuning palm of one of the thousands of homeless who are everywhere around us.

Do you allow yourself to come face-to-face with these unfortunates, or do you turn away from them and your own humanity?

o

ANGUISH AND SELF-DESTRUCTION

I turn on my answering machine and I hear a woman's voice: "Dr. Restak, this is Carol. I called Dan's apartment all day but got no answer. I got frightened and called the police. I was afraid to go over there myself. An officer just called from Dan's. . . . They found him in the apartment. He shot himself."

I barely absorb the rest of the message, the phone number where Carol can be reached, the name of the police officer who wants to talk to me. I'm too busy thinking about Dan, who had been my patient for three years. He was an elderly man with a headache that never seemed to go away, which forever eluded my attempts at diagnosis.

Like waves breaking on a darkened beach, conversational exchanges between Dan and me start washing over me, engulfing me. Certain comments that seemed unremarkable when Dan first made them now took on a dire portentousness in the light of his suicide. "These headaches are really killing me." "I don't know how much more I can take." "Sometimes I feel so bad, I'd do anything to feel better."

The problem wasn't just headaches; they had only been what Dan emphasized most. In addition to the headaches, permeating and interpenetrating them like fog over a coastline, there had been a gripping, unrelenting depression. Unable to free himself from deepening gloom despite endless medications, electroshock therapy, and years of psychiatric treatment, Dan had become withdrawn in recent years. For days at a time he stayed in his apartment, speaking only to Carol, his lady friend, as he referred to her. When the depression and the headaches became too painful to bear, he would call my office and make an appointment.

Three hospitalizations and every test known to medicine failed to reveal a cause for the headaches. Dan and I then concentrated our efforts on the depression, with results that, in the face of Dan's death, were now only too clear.

A patient's suicide takes a double toll on a doctor who sees death and dying as his enemies, proof of his ineptitude or fallibility. Suicide adds an additional burden of guilt. Did I miss something . . . ? Should I have asked him more often whether he was thinking of killing himself . . . ? What if . . . ? Suppose I had . . . ? Would it have helped if I . . . ? Such is the psychiatrist's breviary.

Among the factors that influence a person to enter medicine are the need to be helpful, to make a difference in a patient's life, to care, to comfort, to have one's identity confirmed as a healer. These feelings are all brutalized by a patient's suicide. At such times any doctor worthy of the profession considers temporarily calling it quits, cutting back, cutting down, even cutting out (calling it quits altogether).

These guiltful, blameful ruminations often conceal, as jungle underbrush hides a predator, an implicit assumption that the patient has freely chosen this horrible fate. While most of us would admit considerable reservations about the soundness of mind of a person who chooses death by his own hand, most of us also become incredibly judgmental when the act has actually taken place. Mixed in with that sorrow and guilt, there exists—and don't let any doctor tell you otherwise—an anger so bitter you can almost taste it. The origin of this rage and anger? The physician's sense of failure, of abandonment by the patient for whom death was preferable to another meeting or additional therapeutic exchanges. In retrospect the treatment sessions come to seem as meaningless to the doctor as they must have seemed at the time to the suicide. Make no mistake about it: the successful suicide abandons his doctor; rejects him; expresses in the most public way possible the doctor's irrelevance, anonymity, and psychic impotence. It is a rare doctor who doesn't experience anger as well as sorrow in response to a patient's suicide.

Recent research findings provide some measure of support for the hope that in the very near future, many suicidal patients can be identified ahead of time. A breakdown product of the neurotransmitter serotonin, 5-hydroxyindole acetic acid (5-HIAA), is perceptibly lower in the spinal fluid of successful suicides. This discovery was made by Marie Asberg, a psychiatrist at the Karolinska Hospital and Institute in Stockholm, where patients on the psychiatric wards undergo routine spinal tap (a procedure not usually done on patients in psychiatric hospitals). When the spinal fluids were compared, patients who attempted suicide (successfully or not) were found to have lower levels of 5-HIAA. Among those patients who attempt suicide and survive, 2 percent will try again, this time successfully. But for people with low levels of 5-HIAA and a previous suicide attempt, the figure jumps to 20 percent.

Another group of researchers studied serotonin binding, the tendency for certain brain areas to take up drugs known to bind or attach themselves to the serotonin receptors. This research group was composed of neuroscientists from the Laboratory of Biological Psychiatry, Department of Psychiatry, Case Western Reserve University School of Medicine in Cleveland, Ohio. They discovered that subjects who had committed suicide, compared with people who had died by other means, had a greater number of binding sites in the brain and a greater affinity for serotonin drugs.

Both the Karolinska and the Case Western Reserve work suggest at least implicitly that in the near future, potentially suicidal patients may be identified before they kill themselves. By measuring the contents of spinal fluid or blood, physicians will be able to come up with a marker for suicide potential.

Such prognostic capabilities will usher in a new era in the care and treatment of depressed patients (by far the largest group of suicidal patients). But matters are likely to be more complicated than they first appear. Are there limits beyond which the doctor and others cannot go in the interests of preventing suicide? Specifically, can someone be hospitalized until the 5-HIAA level (or other, yet to be determined metabolic parameter) returns to normal? Suppose the patient no longer feels suicidal, but the 5-HIAA level remains low enough to suggest continued suicidal potential—what then?

And what of patients who never speak of depression, much less of suicide? To prevent such a tragedy, a doctor who suspects the possibility must ask the patient if he feels suicidal and then must take protective measures for the patient's safety. "Suicide tests" will never be able to replace the doctor's capacity to confront and deal with the unthinkable: one person's willingness to destroy by his own hand that which the physician, in common with the majority of mankind, holds to be most dear, life itself.

For all of these reasons, I believe that biological markers for suicidal potential will provide more benefit for doctors than for patients. If tests suggest the possibility of suicide, then the patient could be confined, even against his will; if tests are normal, then everything presently possible has been done to foresee the ultimate calamity. Indeed, it is the doctor's anguish, and not the patient's, that is likely to be assuaged by such tests.

Last night I dreamed about my patient Dan; I hope it will be the last such dream, but I am not confident that it will be. (Even after twenty years I still—though rarely, thank God—dream about Anita, my only other patient who committed suicide.) In the dream I am telling Dan about the new tests, that I want to measure his spinal fluid, that we can help him, and that he doesn't have to take his own life. But in the dream Dan doesn't say anything. He merely looks at me for a moment, smiles enigmatically, then turns away toward the darkness.

o

EVERY
LITTLE MOVEMENT

A sk anyone how to distinguish an animal from a plant, and he or she will start talking to you about movement. Animals move and plants don't (although there are a few curious botanical exceptions). The end product of brain activity in animals is motion, be it as automatic as breathing or as voluntary as reaching to select a book from a shelf. Moreover, without some kind of movement, neither mind nor the presence of life can be reliably determined. At one time observation of the movement of the chest wall was one of the criteria for deciding whether an unresponsive person was living or dead. More sophisticated tests are now available to distinguish life from death, but it's still true that sustained immobility is incompatible with life. That's one of the pleasures of encountering sculpted figures placed in lifelike poses such as can be seen at the curb outside a Washington hotel, where stands a well-dressed businessman in bronze who looks for all the world as if he is hailing a cab. Only his lack of movement proves to us that he's not really alive.

Other examples are the dancers and actors who often appear at conventions dressed up in bizarre outfits and posing without moving a muscle, breathing (or so it seems), blinking, or responding in any way to the spectators' amused and incredulous comments: "Is she alive, or isn't she?" "Is that a statue or a person?"

The motor nervous system, including portions of the brain and the spinal cord with its extended network of motor nerves, is usually seen as parallel to the sensory system, which tells us what is happening in the world: as you detect the tickle produced by a fly on your arm (sensory input), you swat it (motor output). But the organization of the brain and nervous system can't be that simple. A fly can still be accurately located in complete darkness and killed even though it can be neither seen nor, after the disappearance of the initial itch, consciously felt on the surface of the skin. Only an internal representation made by the brain of the body's location in space (schema, as it's referred to by psychologists) could make such a performance possible.

Disturbance in the body's schema can be seen after amputation: the patient complains to the doctor that despite the limb's absence, the "feeling" remains that it is still in place. Less severe but no less bizarre distortions of the body schema occur in the anorexic who, at the extremes of emaciation, may look into a mirror and encounter a fat person. In that case, the disturbed body schema is able to override the evidence of the senses: internal representation dominates over sensory input. But in most instances and with most people, body schema and internal representation remain basically in sync with reality. And when they are, information from the way the body moves can tell us more about a person than anything the individual may do or say. For instance, a trained observer can make important conclusions about personality, mood, and general well-being just by studying a person's gait. Indeed, walking provides a kind of signature in time and space more individuating than anything a person says or does. The psychoanalyst Wilhelm Reich spoke of "character armor."

The obsessive-compulsive's tendency to move stiffly and awkwardly is the motor component of the emotional inhibition that distinguishes this illness. A hysteric's gait is more fluid and bouncy: hips and pelvis swing in a spontaneous and often provocatively insouciant manner. The depressed person moves as slowly and lugubriously as the dark thoughts and somber moods that make his or her world bleak and life seem hardly worth living.

Autistics can now be reliably diagnosed by their distinctive way of walking. The peculiarities of autistic inner life are translated by the brain into specific muscular patterns. These may provide a diagnosis before a word is spoken or even prior to the psychiatrist's learning why this particular patient has been brought for a consultation. These insights are possible only because gait involves both conscious and automatic processes. After the initial decision to move from one place to another, the body moves largely outside conscious awareness. Indeed, few experiences are more inhibiting than conscious attention to the motion of one's feet when walking.

Doctors have long been trying to distinguish conscious, willed components of motion from unconscious processes. Reflex action, for instance, was once considered a purely automatic response that could be studied in isolation from the rest of the brain. Striking the tendon below the kneecap with a reflex hammer produces the knee jerk. What could possibly be more automatic? But as every neurologist knows, a knee jerk can be inhibited by anxiety or by the patient's looking at the knee and concentrating on what's going to happen next. In these cases, the brain, principally the prefrontal cortex, is inhibiting this "spontaneous" reflex.

Other reflexes can also be shown in the laboratory to be far from predictable. If the experimenter progressively increases the intensity of an electric stimulus applied to a decapitated frog's foot, one notices a peculiar progression: first a retraction of the stimulated leg; next a retraction of the opposite leg; finally a retraction of all four legs. Such variations in response depending on the quality of the stimulus hardly suggest hard-wired immutable responses. "The simple reflex is probably a purely abstract conception, because all parts of the nervous system are connected together," writes Nobel Prize–winning neurophysiologist Sir Charles Sherrington. "And no part is probably ever capable of reaction without affecting and being affected by other parts."

One of the consequences of the interconnectedness of the brain and nervous system is that "consciously willed" movements are not easily distinguished from "automatic, unconscious" movements. At certain levels of performance consciously acquired skills become involuntary. A formula 1 racing driver traveling at two hundred miles per hour must react without voluntary intention. The nineteenth-century psychologist William James formulated the issue this way:

> It is a general principle in psychology that consciousness deserts all processes where it could no longer be of use. . . . The marksman ends by thinking of only the exact positions of the goal, the singer only of the perfect sound, the balancer only of the point of the pole whose oscillations he must counteract. The associated mechanism has become so perfect in all these persons that each variation in the thought of the end is functionally correlated with the one movement fitted to bring the latter about. Whilst they were tyros, they thought of their means as well as of their end. . . . But, little by little, they succeeded in dropping all this supernumerary consciousness, and they became secure in their movements exactly in proportion as they did so.

Over the years, athletic performances such as James refers to became separated from intellectual processing, almost as if "real thinking" doesn't involve the body at all. Thinking is a motionless exercise—or so, since Descartes, we've been led to believe. (Rodin's *The Thinker* sits lost in thought and firmly anchored in immobility.) But at some point thought must culminate in action; mere cogitation won't do. The athlete must finally start down the ski slope and not merely think about, visualize, or otherwise fantasize how she is going to go about winning that gold medal. The philosopher must put his thoughts on paper and subject his thinking to the responses of other philosophers, test his thinking on the basis of other philosophers' responses. In all instances mind and thinking must be embodied in some form of action. Not

"I think, therefore I am," as Descartes expressed it, but "I act and by my actions learn who I am." Not "Know thyself," as Socrates advised us, but by movement, and willed action, "Create thyself."

o

DESIGNER
DRUGS

Neuroscientists recently identified a part of the brain important to understanding anxiety. They hope to use this new knowledge to develop drugs that can control or perhaps eliminate anxiety entirely. Despite the enthusiasm about this in scientific circles, I wonder if an anxiety-free society would really be such a good idea.

Anxiety deserves a lot of credit in the evolutionary scheme of things. Without it many of us would not likely even be here. It was anxiety that impelled the prehistoric bush people to startle and bolt in response to unexpected sounds or sudden movements. This heightened startle reaction may not have been a joy to live with, either for its possessor or for those around him, but it increased the likelihood that fright could lead to timely flight, thus providing the opportunity for history's first support group, composed of other survivors of a similarly anxious temperament to laugh and sing around the fire later that evening.

Anxiety serves different and more ambiguous purposes in our own time. We're no longer startled by tigers; lions don't prowl our nation's streets. Our threats these days are mostly interpersonal ones: loss of "face," or control in front of others; lapses of judgment; real or imagined "indignities," or perceived assaults on our self-esteem. Now, I am not claiming that any of these contemporary provocations are any less threatening to a person's well-being than were anxiety-provoking situations in the past. Indeed, they elicit the very same behaviors.

Responding to these perceived threats to our social or psychological integrity, we stock our homes with jars and bottles and vials of anxiety-diminishing agents. Alcohol is the most common, also the least predictable. The same number of drinks that produces an inner calm on Monday can set off an acute agitated anxiety on Tuesday. Heroin and other opiates induce a nirvanalike glow of utter tranquillity and contentment. But when the drug wears off, it feels as though somebody has lifted the top of a skull off so that the whole world could stare at a brain in all its nakedness. With cocaine anxiety is dissipated in a flush of confident buoyancy followed by a thousandfold magnification of what is experienced when, in a nightmare, you step into an empty elevator shaft.

Recently whole new classes of drugs have become popular for anxiety management. All are perfectly legal and, for the most part, don't seem to have serious consequences when taken or in the period after stopping them. They have already accomplished marvelous things for people suffering from emotional disturbances marked by excessive or distorted degrees of anxiety. For instance, one drug, called Inderol, which blocks part of the sympathetic nervous system, is for musicians and others who suffer anxiety when they perform in public. Offstage and when they're not in front of an audience, these performers don't need the drug.

Other people are anxious all the time. In order to function, they require a different sort of antianxiety medication almost around the clock. There are also sufferers from panic states, episodes of intense fear of imminent annihilation accompanied by a rapid heart rate or a feeling of constriction in the chest. Anxiety generated during a panic state can lead to complete social isolation. By staying in the house and away from everything that might set off an anxiety attack, the sufferer achieves some inner peace, but at a great psychological price. A separate class of antianxiety drugs short-circuits this panic-withdrawal reaction. Confidence restored, the person doesn't have to live in dread of another panic attack.

Eliminating anxiety, one of our most basic and primitive internal states, provides the stimulus for tailoring "designer drugs" aimed at exorcising everyone's *personal* demon. Their design will be based on specific studies of blood and spinal fluid and computer-assisted brain wave patterns. Neuropsychological tests will be administered that measure everything from how fast a person can tap his or her fingers to how rapidly he or she can scan a computer-generated display, memorize the contents, and then duplicate the pattern on a screen. Finally, several procedures will be administered in which the subject will be poked and probed by physicians trained in pharmacology, psychiatry, and heaven knows what else. The results of this analysis will determine which drug will be dispensed.

When the designer drug is taken by mouth (perhaps even put under the tongue to increase the rate of absorption), we're promised, some of us will feel better than we ever believed possible.

All of this seems very exciting, but I have some reservations and some questions. What will happen when, after taking our designer drug and experiencing a suitable "glow," we have to go back to the boring office or to the carping mate or to unruly children who hold different agendas for how things should be done? I wonder if the designers of these drugs have given much thought to the real-life effects they will have on us. No matter how good these drugs make us feel, the time will come when we have to face up to what William Faulkner called the eternal verities of love and doubt and sickness. And what about coping with hard work, boredom, and the uncertainty about how to get through one's day? Somehow I don't think there's ever going to be a designer drug to handle these kinds of things. My concern is that designer drugs will lead to the same behavioral patterns of every other mood- and behavior-altering drug: withdrawal, self-absorption, a lack of concern about anything other than what's happening inside the user's own head. "Tune in, turn on, drop out," as Timothy Leary put it in the old LSD days. Or, in more contemporary terms, "If the world isn't behaving as you believe that it should, and you feel good while taking your own special drug, then say no to the world rather than to the drug."

Thanks to our desire to be permanently rid of anxiety, even anxiety that may be helpful if we can only tune in to it, we might one day find ourselves desperately alone except for our designer drugs. That experience should stir up some anxiety. But recognizing it may take some moments, because by that time, anxiety may not have been experienced in several years. At that point, if we're lucky, most of us may then consider its return to be not such a bad experience after all. If we're even smarter and luckier, we may have the good sense to toss our designer drugs into the trash and out of our lives.

THE CREATIVITY OF THE UNCONSCIOUS

I once asked Anthony Burgess about his method of "aleatory composition: directing one's plot according to words chosen at hazard from a reference book."

I had two reasons for asking. First, I found it difficult to believe that a random method could provide the basis for Burgess's complex, powerful works; second, I wondered if this total trusting in luck (deriving from *alea* and *aleatory*, the Latin for dice and dice player) could give me important insights into a subject of current interest: creativity and the human brain.

Burgess confirmed that he did use this method and that he believed aleatory composition freed up certain creative tensions that would otherwise remain unexpressed. He suggested that if I had any doubt about the method's effectiveness, I should try it myself. He was pleased, as well as surprised, by my inquiry, because it was based on a comparatively obscure reference he had made several years earlier in a review in the *Times Literary Supplement*.

Some months later I encountered a second reference to the aleatory approach. Edward de Bono, a physician and expert in creativity, called the process "provocation," the introduction of a random word. "The word can be picked from a dictionary with a table of random numbers so that no unconscious selection takes place. Does this mean that any word whatsoever may be used as a provocation with any problem whatsoever? It does. There is no connection (logical) at all between the random word and the problem." De Bono referred to his method as "lateral thinking"; its purpose, he said, was "to produce ideas that are logical in hindsight."

Burgess's and de Bono's emphasis on chance and serendipity turns the creative process upside down. The writer or the problem solver no longer functions as a master technician, consciously aiming the thinking process in a certain direction for a certain set purpose. Now the role becomes that of a gambler who, being dealt a certain hand, must decide on a creative course of action with those cards and only those cards. Both techniques aim at altering perceptions and concepts via the introduction of unexpected, bizarre, and even disorienting associations.

Studies of patients who have undergone "split brain" operations (the separation of the right and left hemispheres) reveal the right hemisphere is superior to its counterpart on the left when it comes to coping with the novel and unfamiliar. This is especially true when there are no clues how to respond. Both aleatory composition and provocation shift the emphasis from the logical—verbal—linear processing style of the left hemisphere to the more holistic style of the right hemisphere, in which logical analysis plays a much smaller part. The right hemisphere may thus be viewed as a "jack of all trades, a generalist that addresses new problems without preconceptions and tries many approaches to a problem until it finds one that fits," according to one summary of right and left hemisphere functioning.

At the anatomical level, the right hemisphere is uniquely suited for creativity, since it occupies a larger volume in the "association cortex," where the most complex levels of information processing and integration are carried out. Second, the right hemisphere contains many long fibers that connect widely separated regions; the left hemisphere, in contrast, contains shorter fibers that provide richer interconnections *within* a specific region.

Innovative drawing and writing techniques and suggestions for improving one's productivity in business and finance are only some of the fields influenced by the introduction of "right brain thinking" over the past decade.

But one must be careful of oversimplifications. The brain always works as a unit; therefore, to imply that in the ordinary person the right hemisphere can somehow be separated from the left is inaccurate and misleading. This organization unifies the personality and precludes abrupt and disorienting discoveries about oneself.

For instance, in a split brain patient, feelings can be aroused by events perceived by the right hemisphere. An explanation for these feelings, however, becomes difficult, if not impossible, because the left hemisphere isn't privy to the experience responsible for the feelings. In a famous experiment of neuroscientist Michael Gazzaniga, a picture of a scantily clad woman is projected to the right hemisphere, and the subject blushes and stammers. When asked, "Why are you blushing?" the subject says, "Oh, doctor, sometimes you do things that are so funny." The true reason for the blushing and stammering isn't available to consciousness.

How different this is from the "unconscious work" that provides a basis for creative expression. In 1912 the German poet Rainer Maria Rilke abruptly stopped writing in the middle of his long poem the "Duino Elegies." Despite his best efforts to continue with it, Rilke found what he called "utterance and release" in another poem, the "Sonnets to Orpheus." Within three weeks he finished the "Duino Elegies," along with 1,200 lines of concentrated, intricately crafted poetry that he wrote down in first draft almost as if he were taking dictation. Rilke could not explain the source of his creativity, but the groundwork had been set over the years by his sustained creative efforts.

Another example of unconscious creativity is the work of the chemist Friedrich August Kekule, who discovered the structure of the benzene ring in a dream. The foundation for the dream was prepared years earlier when Kekule, then a student, testified before a grand jury investigating the cause of a neighbor's death. Among the deceased's effects was a gold ring made in the shape of two intertwined snakes biting their own tails—the alchemical symbol of the unity and variability of matter. Fifteen years later that ring influenced Kekule, who was pondering the mystery of the arrangement of benzene's six carbon and six hydrogen atoms.

"One night," Kekule wrote in his diary, "I turned my chair to the fire and sank into a doze." He dreamed of atoms swirling and dancing, joining together and then pulling apart in a motion that finally settled into a snakelike pattern. At that moment, "one of the serpents caught its own tail and the ring thus formed whirled exasperatingly before my eyes. I awoke as by lightning and spent the rest of the night working out the logical consequences of the hypothesis."

When he awakened, Kekule suggested that the benzene molecule is a six-layered structure consisting of carbon atoms from which hydrogen atoms are suspended like charms from a bracelet. The signet ring stimulated the creative visualization. This randomly chosen image, the aleatory component, led to the artful depiction and solution of one of nature's mysteries. Kekule's insights could not have been forced any more than Rilke could have forced the "Duino Elegies."

For both Kekule and Rilke the creative process demanded a surrender of a logical, everyday modus operandi based on deductions, "sticking to the facts," and strictly logical reasoning.

It's useful to think of creativity as borrowing more from the right than the left hemisphere, but such an ordering is only metaphorical. The *whole brain,* as mentioned previously, is involved in creativity, the two hemispheres communicating with each other over eight hundred million neurofibers. The vast network of the human brain contains two hundred billion neural cells, each connected with anywhere from one thousand to ten thousand other cells, creating the potential for any one cell to influence a distant other through any number of intervening connections. This possibility for long-range interconnectivity provides the physical framework for the aleatory method mentioned by Anthony Burgess. A randomly chosen word is linked via the creative process with a thought that, if the effort is truly creative, has never been thought before. The process is similar to the discovery of previously un-suspected linkages among neurons within the brain. In such a process the brain provides a means for creativity, while at the same time the creative product (the work of art or a ground-breaking scientific insight) mirrors the operation of the brain from which it originates.

Indeed, creativity is hauntingly similar to the brain in which it is embedded. The closer we seek to examine and understand cre-ativity and the brain, the more opaque they become. It would take a poet with a deep knowledge of the brain to capture something like this in words. Sir Charles Sherrington came the closest:

It is as if the Milky Way entered upon some cosmic dance. Swiftly the brain becomes an enchanted loom where millions of flashing shuttles weave a dissolving pattern, always a meaningful pattern, although never an abiding one; a shifting harmony of subpatterns.

o

KICKING
THE HABIT

I t's three weeks now since my last cigarette. I think I finally
got this thing licked."
        An instant of eye contact confirms that . . . yes, this thirty-
five-year-old woman is perfectly serious in asserting, after
only three weeks of abstinence, that she has overcome ten years of
smoking.

If a gambler had been at our table at that moment, he could have
made a killing. My friend was so convinced she had licked her
smoking habit, she would have bet a lot of money that she would
never smoke another cigarette. It would have been a very risky
wager, because the odds were not at all in her favor. Only 20
percent of those who have sworn off cigarettes are still nonsmokers
at the end of a year because the nicotine component of tobacco
creates a craving and physical dependence. A 1986 report from the
Harvard School of Public Health states, "Nicotine has a profile of
behavioral and physiologic effects typical of other drugs of abuse
and, like the heroin derived from opium, meets rigorous experimental criteria as a drug with considerable potential to cause
dependence."

Any substance that creates dependence—opium, nicotine, alcohol, cocaine, or marijuana—does so by exerting direct pharma-
cologic effects on the brain, specifically on those areas involved in
mood. Why are so many of us reaching out for mood-altering sub-

stances? This Big Question is unanswerable, because every individual who gets hooked on tobacco and other substances of abuse has a different reason for doing so. The next most important area of inquiry relates to the brain mechanisms involved in tobacco addiction. One thing is immediately apparent: addiction doesn't occur with that first cigarette; most smokers experience nausea, sometimes even vomiting, the first time they light up. But if they repeat the experience again and again, several highly pleasurable and reinforcing effects soon start to be associated with tobacco. Included among them are increased alertness, improved and more sustained attention, diminished aggression and irritability, and decreased appetite, leading to weight loss.

Smarter, less stressed, less aggressive, thinner, more focused and concentrated—if nicotine can make us all of these things, then it is a wonder that all of us aren't compulsive smokers. One of the reasons we are not is that nobody enjoys the experience of becoming dependent on something. We like to think we can accomplish on our own all the good things that tobacco can do for us. Add to that the health warnings against tobacco and the videotaped-before-death messages of actors exhorting us from beyond the grave not to smoke. Clearly the much-publicized drop in the percentage of people who continue to smoke makes good sense. Nobody wants to die of cancer or heart disease, to mention just two potential health consequences from smoking. But like all other addictions, addiction to tobacco isn't a rational thing; some of us continue to do what we know is downright harmful to us.

This paradox becomes understandable if we think of tobacco addiction as a brain disease rather than as evidence of moral weakness or character deficiency. The brain contains certain receptors for the neurotransmitter acetylcholine, which mediates a whole host of brain processes, including pleasure. Nicotine occupies these receptors quite comfortably. With each inhalation of tobacco, these processes become linked with nicotine, and physical dependence follows. The withdrawal syndrome produces craving, sleeplessness, nervousness, increased appetite, and mood changes. The brain seems to function at its sharpest only in response to a steady supply of nicotine. Cut off that supply, and one irrational part of the body longs for something that another, more rational part has set itself against.

For the longest time, I thought this internal war was an unmitigated disaster, a schism within the psyche from which no good could possibly come. I am not so convinced of that now. For one thing, a continued battle against tobacco—or other substances of abuse, for that matter—introduces some things back into our lives that are missing in the frenetic life-style that most of us are caught up in. To kick the tobacco habit, a person must direct sustained attention and concentration upon a single goal; take the long view rather than the short, "quick fix" approach; get his or her own personal "act" together; and, finally, gain insight into himself or herself as vulnerable but ultimately self-determining. Anything that stimulates and enhances us so positively can't be all bad. One could even make the case, I suppose, although I don't go quite that far myself, that a person may be better off for the experience of having been at one time substance-dependent.

This "happy to have been hooked" orientation can be observed among members of antismoking and other support groups. For the first time in their lives, some of these people have accomplished something they are really proud of. Their lives now have meaning: "I was torn apart by this chemical, but now, thanks to my own efforts and the help of the other members of this group, I am whole again. Hallelujah."

But as with all conversions, redemption must be followed by a constant vigilance lest the transgressor slip back into the old ways. That statistic of 20 percent abstinence at the end of one year reminds us that the war never really ends and that the good soldier must fight on one day at a time.

After thinking all this over, I am not about to tell my friend that she is on the short end of the odds in regard to quitting her smoking. After three weeks she is still hanging in, determined to break a habit that, if it lasts long enough, will surely break her.

Granted, her efforts to stop smoking aren't glamorous or heroic. Nor are they aspects of the good life most of us are taught to pursue. But her resolve and vigilance to reject a substance of proven destructiveness will enhance her self-esteem and extend her life— prizes well worth the battle she is waging.

○

YOUR BRAIN HAS
A MIND OF ITS OWN

At the moment of decision we all feel we are acting freely, selecting at will from an infinity of choices.

Yet recent research suggests this sense of freedom may be merely an illusory by-product of the way the human brain operates.

Consider something as simple as your decision to read this essay. You quickly scan the title and a few phrases here and there until, at a certain moment, you make the mental decision to read on. You then focus on the first paragraph and begin to read.

The internal sequence was always thought to be: 1. you make a conscious decision to read; 2. that decision triggers your brain into action; 3. your brain then signals the hands to stop turning pages, focuses the eyes on the paragraph, and so on.

But new findings indicate that a very different process actually takes place. An inexplicable but plainly measurable burst amount of activity occurs in your brain prior to your conscious desire to act. An outside observer monitoring electrical fluctuations in your brain can anticipate your action about a third of a second before you are aware that you have decided to act.

That sequence was observed by Benjamin Libet, a neurophysiologist at the School of Medicine of the University of California at San Francisco. His experiment has raised intriguing and disturbing questions about whether our intentions may be more determined and predictable than we realize (or would like to admit).

In Libet's experiment each subject is outfitted with a number of on-scalp electrodes that detect the changing voltage potentials of underlying brain activity. The subject is then asked to flex his forefinger briskly at any time he chooses. The procedure is designed to eliminate any possibility of suggestion by the experimenter or any other factor that might influence the timing of the decision. It is an optimal free-choice situation.

As part of the experiment, measurements are taken of brain activity preceding the self-initiated movement. The recordings reveal that the subjects first make up their minds to move at about two hundred milliseconds (a fifth of a second) before the actual movement. The subjects themselves verify the timing of that instant by matching the moment of their decision to the position of a dot of light revolving around a clock face.

But Libet's electrodes detect a sudden flurry of brain activity that arises, on average, 350 milliseconds (about a third of a second) *before* the subjects' *conscious* choice. "The brain 'decides' to initiate or at least to prepare to initiate the act before there is any reportable subjective awareness that such a decision has taken place," says Libet.

At first glance this conclusion seems paradoxical, improbable, even absurd. We usually experience our decisions as freely emanating from an "I" or a "self," a center of command. But Libet's findings contradict that: the brain is actually in operation before our conscious act of will. "Cerebral initiation even of a spontaneous voluntary act of the kind studied here can and usually does begin unconsciously," says Libet. (The term "unconscious," as he employs it, refers not to the Freudian/psychological concept, but simply to processes that are not experienced consciously.)

Libet's research touches on one of mankind's oldest conundrums: Do we possess a free will, or are we governed by inexorable determinism?

Central to this puzzle is the pivotal role we assign to consciousness. Consciously we experience ourselves as the conscious initiators of all that we do. But despite the emphasis that we place on consciousness, mental life can and usually does proceed quite nicely without it. Would you really want to be fully conscious of all the minute muscular activities involved in holding this book? Instead, your consciousness is focused on what you are now reading.

A century ago in *The Principles of Psychology* William James pinpointed self-reference as the basis upon which consciousness rests. "The universal conscious fact is not 'feelings exist' and 'thoughts exist,' but 'I think' and 'I feel.' " Who is this "I," and where does he live? Until recently there was no way of scientifically answering that question. Consciousness could be experienced, but it evaded objective demonstration. During the nineteenth century psychologists did the best they could under the circumstances. They had trained observers use introspection to investigate perceptions, memories, thoughts, and feelings. But as Freud revealed, our conscious mental lives are only a veneer beneath which lies a chaos of impulses, emotions, and motives.

In our own time the study of consciousness took a new and fascinating turn with the use of sophisticated computers to collect and collate the electrical impulses generated by the brain. One of the wave forms recorded was the "readiness potential."

In the late 1960s researchers discovered that the readiness potential begins about a second before a voluntary act. But when, scientists asked themselves, does the instant of conscious intent occur? And can it be measured?

Now, thanks to Libet's findings, we are beginning to answer those questions—and, in the process, to cast doubt on the seemingly obvious proposition that conscious intention is the initial event, after which everything else falls into place.

The discovery will seem less paradoxical if we can free ourselves from the preconception that the mind, the "I," is somehow separate from the brain, and that the relationship between the two is that of a commanding officer to a subordinate. Research data simply do not support that model. In the words of brain researcher Eric

Hearth, "the power of determining one's own behavior is not the power of one entity (the mind) over another (the body), but the influence that the brain has on itself."

Moreover, contemporary research indicates that there is no single center in the brain involved with the experience of will. Rather, will and other expressions of the mind are distributed functions, occurring in many locations at once. "Whenever motor acts or perceptions have been properly analyzed, they have been found to have involved large numbers of neurons in different parts of the brain," says Nobel Prize–winning neurophysiologist Ragnar Granit. "For this reason, it also seems likely that conscious awareness as a process necessarily implicates a vast number of cells from different centers."

At different times and under different circumstances we are more or less conscious, act more or less intentionally. Think of the dimming of the house lights in a movie theater just before the show. People become aware of the dimming at different moments, depending on what they're doing—talking to a companion, eating popcorn, glancing around, and so on. But the process always progresses from an initial uncertainty about the change in illumination to a fully conscious conviction that the lights are indeed going out.

A similar pattern prevails in regard to will. In most instances our decisions are gradual ones in the middle of a continuum between instant, impulsive actions and agonizing indecisiveness.

Subliminal-perception experiments provide additional evidence that consciousness and will are emergent processes, appearing only gradually once neuronal interaction reaches a certain level of complexity. For example, if an experimenter flashes words on a screen at a rate too fast to be read, subjects will exhibit different time thresholds for recognizing that they have seen different kinds of words. Usually they take longer to identify taboo or threatening words than they do to identify less emotionally charged terms. Why the difference? The brain may be analyzing meaning and as a result modifying its own level of arousal to hasten or retard awareness of the information. In essence, the brain analyzes the words for their emotional significance, as well as for semantic features and patterns, before they reach consciousness.

Where, then, is free will in all of this? Do Libet's findings render us mere automatons? Are we slaves to our own brains? Is our sense of freedom nothing but a face-saving illusion? Not quite.

Libet has learned that his subjects can "veto" their decisions during the one-tenth to two-tenths of a second between their first awareness of intent and the action itself. (Outside the laboratory similar last-moment changes of mind frequently take place. On the way home from work you may suddenly, at the last moment, choose a slightly longer but more scenic route after you had already "made up your mind" to take the short one.) This ability to cancel the brain's decision is, in Libet's opinion, the bedrock upon which rests individual responsibility and free will.

"Although the volitional process may be initiated by unconscious cerebral activity," he says, "conscious control of the actual motor performance of voluntary acts definitely remains possible. The findings should, therefore, be taken not as being antagonistic to free will, but rather as affecting the view of how free will must operate."

According to that model, free will operates via the selection and control of intentions that, for the most part, arise spontaneously. "The thought comes when 'it' will, not when 'I' will," was how Friedrich Nietzsche described the process one hundred years ago in *Beyond Good and Evil*.

If intentions arise spontaneously, as Libet's experiments clearly imply, then actions rather than thoughts or "temptations" are our chief form of self-definition. That is, we are what we do rather than what we think, fantasize, or otherwise inwardly experience about ourselves.

The ramifications for moral philosophy are extremely intriguing. If free will exists chiefly in veto power over spontaneously arising intentions, then it is hardly surprising that so many moral and ethical directives are formulated so as to emphasize the importance of inhibition. Most of the Ten Commandments, for instance, are phrased as prohibitions. The intentions of Judeo-Christian religion and the findings of neurophysiology are in agreement on the nature of the will.

"The concept of conscious veto or blockage of the motor performance of specific intentions to act," says Libet, "is in general accord with certain religious and humanistic views of ethical behavior and individual responsibility. 'Self-control' of the acting-out of one's intentions is commonly advocated; in the present terms, this would operate by conscious selection or control of whether the unconsciously initiated final volitional process will be implemented in action."

Such a view lends little support to the Socratic dictum "Know thyself." Rather, the emphasis on action agrees more closely with the doctrine of Danish philosopher Søren Kierkegaard: "Choose thyself." We are truly ourselves only when we act. "We may start with the proposition that the only direct outward effects of our will are bodily movements," wrote William James in 1890 in the *Principles*.

Contemporary brain research thus suggests that over the centuries, philosophers and psychologists have been asking the wrong question: How does the mind, through the exercise of will, operate on the brain? Will, it now appears, is intrinsically related to brain activity. At the most fundamental level, each brain has a mind of its own.

THE FICTION
OF THE
REASONABLE MAN

The actions of Bernhard Goetz were not those of a reasonable person."

A lawyer said that to me at a dinner party at the time of the trial of Bernhard Goetz, the "subway vigilante" accused of shooting four teenagers he stated were about to attack him.

Another dinner guest added: "The jury is going to have to examine the circumstances under which every bullet was fired and ask themselves, 'Was this the behavior of a reasonable person?' If there's any indication that even one of those shots was unnecessary, Goetz should be found guilty."

What they were referring to was the ruling by New York State's Court of Appeals in July of 1986 that a claim of self-defense (such as Goetz had made against charges of attempted murder and assault) must be judged by the dual standard of "reasonableness." During the trial the jurors were asked to determine not only that Goetz subjectively believed that he was acting reasonably, but that on an objective level his actions were those any "reasonable man" would pursue in the same circumstances.

As a neurologist and neuropsychiatrist with over a decade of experience in conducting pretrial interviews of individuals who have acted violently, I believe the "reasonable person" argument an illogical and outdated approach to fully understanding events in the Goetz case and other selective instances of violence. On the basis of what I know about the human brain, I'm convinced that no one acts reasonably when feeling threatened by death or severe bodily harm.

Deep within every reasonable person's brain is the limbic system, an ancient interconnected network of structures that anatomically and chemically have changed little over hundreds of thousands of years. We share these structures with jungle animals, as well as animals that many reasonable people keep as pets. Under conditions of extreme duress the limbic system is capable of overwhelming the cerebral cortex, wherein many of the reasonable person's most reasonable attributes—like interpretation, judgment, and restraint—are formulated.

The limbic system (from the Latin *limbus*, meaning border or seam) lies along the margin of the cerebral cortex and includes the amygdala, hippocampus, and other components, which interact directly with the thalamus and hypothalamus below. Taken together, they govern aggressive behavior.

Malfunctions in the system or its various neurotransmitters (chemicals that relay signals among brain parts) can cause temporarily deranged behavior. Such behavior can be chemically induced with such compounds as PCP ("angel dust"), which acts on the hippocampus and induces impulsive behavior; or it can be suppressed with drugs such as lithium, which boosts the level of a ' neurotransmitter called serotonin, important in the reduction of aggression.

In most instances the limbic system is an asset. Without it, few of our ancestors would have survived to enable us to be here asserting our reasonableness.

Occasionally the limbic system can malfunction because of a pathological condition, such as a tumor, or for other reasons still unknown. It overwhelms rationality, resulting in panic attacks, outbursts of rage, perhaps even murder.

• An executive on his way to an important business meeting begins to experience chest pain, shortness of breath, an agonizing feeling that he's about to die. A special brain test known as a PET scan reveals in vivid color an area of heightened activity within the limbic system. With tranquilizer medication the "panic attack" subsides, leaving the executive embarrassed and frightened that he could have so suddenly "lost control."

• Epileptic discharges deep within the limbic system are detected in a thirty-five-year-old man charged with murder. He claims that he cannot recall the murder. Witnesses state that the man suddenly broke into a violent rage during which the murder occurred. Did epilepsy make him lose control? A psychiatrist is prepared to testify that it did on the basis of an electroencephalogram showing epileptic discharges in the anterior temporal lobe.

In the 1950s neurosurgeons discovered that if parts of the limbic system are electrically stimulated during a brain operation, the patient will experience fear and panic. Specific chemicals can cause the same reactions in certain individuals. A patient given to panic attacks is hooked up to an intravenous feeder. Within a few minutes after starting an infusion of sodium lactate solution, a commonly administered fluid replacement, a limbic-based attack of sudden overwhelming fear takes over. Despite his best efforts the patient is unable to calm himself. But after the lactate solution is stopped and a tranquilizer administered, the limbic discharge subsides and the patient calms down.

Many brain scientists are convinced that the limbic system may also be responsible for sudden outbursts of rage followed by violence—the so-called episodic dyscontrol syndrome. Limbic involvement has not appeared in every such patient, but enough cases have turned up with limbic abnormalities to warrant the use of electroencephalograms and other neurologic tests in cases of seemingly inexplicable outbursts of violence.

These discoveries linking some cases of violence to electrical discharges in the limbic system have important implications for any comprehensive theory about human behavior. Emotions are not incidental and subsidiary to rational processes. Even at his or her most reasonable moments, and despite all best efforts to the contrary, a person remains strongly influenced by feelings and emotions. (Psychologist William James described the interpenetration of thought and feeling long before the limbic system was discovered in an aptly titled essay, "The Sentiment of Rationality.")

Our legal system, however, has yet to incorporate these new insights: the reasonable man standard continues to be stressed. But as Guido Calabresi, dean of Yale Law School, points out in his book *Ideals, Beliefs, Attitudes and the Law*, definitions of "reasonable" have varied according to different cultures. In Roman law it was *bonus paterfamilias*, "the good father of the family"; in England, "the man on the Clapham omnibus"—something like your typical subway rider. In the United States, a typical definition given by courts and commentators is "the man who takes the magazines at home and in the evening pushes the lawn mower in his shirtsleeves."

Common to all of these descriptions has been the ordinariness and predictability of the "reasonable" person. But in the last century two major developments have occurred that make those criteria less valid. The first was the work of Sigmund Freud, whose description of the unconscious suggested that forces outside a person's control could exert a powerful influence on behavior. The insanity defense, with all its ramifications and variations, is based on this premise. That's why psychiatrists and not criminologists have traditionally testified, frequently offering conflicting opinions, as to whether a defendant is responsible for his actions.

The second development, sociobiology, arrived in the 1970s. According to sociobiologists, selection pressures exerted by the natural and social environments favor one behavior over another. Many of those behaviors are genetically determined. Over the past two decades genetic factors have been found to exert a strong influence on such mental illnesses as schizophrenia and manic depression. These agents modify the expression of certain personality disorders, such as obsessions and compulsions, and even influence such normal personality traits, as shyness or extroversion. An individual's actions, reasonable or otherwise, are therefore considered within the context of genes, environment, and surrounding society.

Currently the neurosciences have provided even more dramatic information about the role played by the limbic system. Consider this description, written by the subject's psychiatrist, of a fifty-one-year-old man who suddenly went into a tantrum because his wife and children differed with him on a trivial family matter: "Rage would well up within him, and he would begin cursing at the top of his voice. The feeling was one of lack of control, and soon he would begin smashing windows, breaking up the furniture, putting his fist through the walls and doors. This could go on for hours. He was aware of what was happening but felt driven to continue."

Except for these rare episodes, this man is otherwise indistinguishable from other family men who work regularly in middle-management positions. Do his outbursts reflect some form of "temporary insanity"? Or is he a reasonable man who becomes temporarily *un*reasonable? Whatever the answer, his outbursts— diagnosed by his psychiatrist as episodes of limbic dysfunction— are notable for two qualities. Once aroused to fury, the man feels "driven to continue," and the episodes can "go on for hours."

Given what we now know of such cases, the logic of the reasonable man standard in the Bernhard Goetz case, or similar cases in the future, may be inherently flawed.

"We don't contend that the defendant had no cause for apprehension," said Assistant District Attorney Gregory Waples on the first day of the trial. He argued that Goetz, once aroused, should have been capable of stopping himself at one point. His firing of a second shot into one of the assailants, Darrell Cabey, after, as the prosecution has contended, the immediate threat was over, is crucial to the state's argument. "When [Goetz] fired that last shot," Waples said, "beyond the slightest doubt, Cabey was seated, helpless, doing nothing to threaten or menace Bernhard Goetz." Consequently, according to Waples, Goetz is open to the charge that he did not act as a reasonable person.

The prosecutor's logic is that once Goetz coolly discerned that he was out of danger, he should have calmed down, put away his gun, and awaited the arrival of the police.

Although this undoubtedly would have made things easier for Goetz, such expectations are neurologically unrealistic. Once aroused, the limbic system can become a directive force for hours, sometimes days, and can rarely be shut off as if by flipping a switch. The heart keeps pounding; harsh and labored breathing burns in the throat; fear is replaced by anger and, finally, murderous rage. At some point in this process memories for ongoing events may become permanently lost; false memories may be created as the frightened and enraged person repeatedly relives the violent act he committed in response to what he perceived as a threat to his life.

Consider Goetz's response to the question "Did you just shoot each one of these people just once?"

Goetz: "Well, you see that's why I . . . that's . . . that's one of the things that puzzles me. . . . Because you know what you're doing, you cannot do something and not know it. I mean, how could I do it and not know it? But if you can accept this, I was out of control, and that's . . . you know . . . but that's . . . that's . . . it's true. Maybe you should always be in control, but if you . . . if you put people in a situation where they're threatened with mayhem, several times, and then if . . . then if something happens, and if a person acts, turns into a vicious animal . . . That's not the end of the shooting. That's what . . . It's not the end. I ran back to the first two, to make sure."

Is that what a *reasonable* person would do under such circumstances?

Lawyers and judges love to explore such questions, but I'm convinced that these are the wrong questions. They reflect an outmoded orientation that overemphasizes the intellect. Excluded are the deep and powerful emotional currents of fear, self-preservation, or territoriality that can surface in any one of us and overpower our ability to reason.

This may not be a pretty or elegant arrangement, but as long as our brain is organized the way it is, none of us should be too confident that we would remain completely reasonable if we perceived our life to be in imminent danger. This critical perception of threat isn't based on rationality. It's fueled by those limbic-derived emotions that have ensured the survival of our species.

Isn't it preferable, therefore, to face up courageously to these sometimes frightening and unpleasant realities? Shouldn't we stop pretending that questions such as those asked about Bernhard Goetz can be answered by courtroom speculations about how a reasonable person would have responded in his place?

To expect reasonable behavior in the face of perceived threat, terror, and rage is itself a most unreasonable expectation.

o

INFORMATION OVERLOAD

Studying the complexities of the human brain makes you realize that, no matter how hard you try, you can never learn everything about it. The vast amount of available information overwhelms one's mental resources—registration, comprehension, memory retention, retrieval, recall—so that after a while the mind simply gives up trying to take it all in.

Nor is information overload confined to students of the brain. We are all inundated with more facts and information than we can possibly absorb, often on trivial subjects we care nothing about. For instance, twenty-four-hour news stations repeat trifling events over and over again throughout the day and night just to fill up air time. After the third or fourth repetition we just hear the sounds of the words without really absorbing their sense.

Just how much information about the weather does a person really need in order to decide whether to take an umbrella to the office? Yet weather reports are now provided by meteorologists who spew forth detailed information about atmospheric conditions comprehensible and of interest only to other meteorologists.

A lady friend suffering from information overload (but who so far hasn't been diagnosed, much less treated for her disorder) routinely keeps three televisions running in the morning so that she can monitor all three network morning news programs and "not miss anything important." Her husband, a print information junkie, sits at the breakfast table rapidly scanning three newspapers as the TV channels blare essentially the same story.

I also know several information bulimics who go on weekend binges reading dozens of magazines they've accumulated. They eagerly stuff themselves with a huge supply of facts that they later disgorge at cocktail parties to friends and strangers alike. Nor do I believe it entirely coincidental that a game like Trivial Pursuit, which emphasizes one's skill in remembering massive amounts of truly trivial information, once so captured our national imagination. But such tendencies are everywhere in our society. Mention a movie or a book during a casual conversation with an information junkie, and immediately you will be given the names of all the extras in the movie or told that the typeface used for the book was Monotype Perpetua. At such times I wonder, Just how much more information can the brain possibly deal with?

The short answer to that question is that the processing capacity of the human brain regulates how much information we can take in over a given period of time. The nineteenth-century psychologist Hermann Ebbinghaus discovered while memorizing nonsense syllables (daf, dak, klim, and so on) that a mathematical relationship exists between the number of repetitions made on a given day and the rapidity and accuracy of repeating the list on the following day. These principles of information processing are based on the organization of the brain. Once limits on the brain's capacity are exceeded, symptoms of information overload appear: failures of response; irritability; boredom; the inability to take decisive action (there are simply too many variables to keep track of); finally, a pervading sense of "so what?" The affected individual, particularly in a moderately advanced case, starts taking actions that would have seemed unthinkable only a few weeks earlier. Magazine and newspaper subscriptions are canceled; radios and TVs unplugged; conversations modified to avoid at all costs giving out or taking in too many facts. At this point in the illness, information is disorienting and confusing; it subtracts from, rather than adds to, one's competence.

The fact is that much of the "authoritative" information that we're given tends over the long run to be inconsistent and maddeningly contradictory. For instance, a year or so ago experts encouraged us to drink moderate amounts of alcohol daily. This practice seemed to correlate positively with increased longevity. Within months of that advice, however, other, equally respected researchers questioned the advice on the grounds that some latent alcoholics may, as a result of daily drinking, slip into alcoholism. Besides, they added, a woman of childbearing age who might be getting pregnant any time soon should avoid alcohol completely. The fetus could be damaged during the first few weeks before a woman even knows that she is pregnant. *What* is one to do with such conflicting bits of information?

Take jogging as another example. A decade ago jogging enthusiasts, many of them medical people, assured us that in contrast to just about everything else in life, jogging needn't be practiced in moderation. The more jogging you do, the healthier you'll be—that was the general message. Now, in the wake of deaths while running and numerous cases of heart attack, stress fracture, and torn cartilage, many health experts put down jogging and suggest vigorous walking instead.

As a result of such information turnabouts, many of us, who suffer the pangs of advanced information disease, are saying, however illogically, "Enough already. Don't confuse me with any more facts."

Junk foods provide a good metaphor for this concept. Much of the information bombarding us from our televisions and radios lacks redeeming nutritional value, dulls our sensibilities, and leaves us idea-wise, bloated with trivia yet at the same time intellectually deprived. In short, too much nonessential news about nonevents may be hazardous to our mental health.

What's needed are techniques aimed at freeing us from useless information that, like atherosclerotic plaque, plugs our creative circuits and infarcts our ideas. We must develop some new vital reflex for our self-protection and self-regulation. Illiteracy may be such a reflex. Not the familiar illiteracy of being unable to read or write, but rather a more limited, voluntary, and "enlightened" illiteracy, an *unwillingness* to read about subjects that we really don't *need* to know anything about.

The growing mountain of information facing us these days makes higher and more enlightened forms of illiteracy extremely desirable. What will they be like? Perhaps one will be new fitness and vacation facilities.

Imagine a spa, a "fat farm," somewhere in the Southwest. But this facility operates a bit differently. The "fat" that people have come to the spa to shed is informational, not physical: the plethora of facts and knowledge carried around on subjects that the bearer cares little or nothing about. In self-defense—and for a lot of money—all of us in the not-so-distant future may be attending such a spa. Once there, we'll relax in a dark, soundproofed room, not reading, hearing, or speaking about anything.

At the end of our stay in this futuristic mind spa, we'll join our fellow participants in a group discussion session. Accompanied by cheers and encouragement, the members will discourse proudly on everything they *don't* know or care in the least to learn anything about.

o

WHEN IGNORANCE IS BLISS

I magine that you know you have a fifty–fifty chance of coming down in twenty years with an incurable brain disease that will make you insane, then kill you. Suppose a medical test was currently available that would tell you with absolute certainty what your fate would be. Would you choose to take the test? Would you want your children to take the test?

These are not hypothetical questions. Technological advances permit us to make such predictions. Using available tests, patients with seemingly everyday physical or emotional problems may be diagnosed to be on the road, years from now, to a full-blown, devastating case of multiple sclerosis, manic depression, Alzheimer's disease, or schizophrenia. I've come to think that this new ability to peer into the future places physicians and patients in an unprecedented paradoxical position; in certain instances, the less both of them know, the better off they may be. Discovering the future at the cost of ruining the good years a person at risk may still have to enjoy might be a Faustian bargain at best.

For example, not long ago I encountered an old enemy hidden within the brain of a forty-three-year-old man who came to my office to discuss a problem with his memory. His wife accompanied him and sat there tense and frightened while I completed my examination.

The man was right. His memory was failing; so, too, were his judgment, his temper, his mood, and, little by little, his self-respect. But it wasn't until I saw a brief, sudden, jarring movement of his body—almost as if the building had been rocked by a small earthquake—that I knew what was wrong. He suffered from Huntington's chorea.

While still a resident, I encountered my first patient with that disease. He, too, was dimly aware that he was losing his mind. First there had been temper tantrums. Over a period of time they were followed by memory problems and jerking movements. Insanity and then, mercifully, death ended this man's agony.

My recent patient was also in an early stage in the illness, and to tell the truth, that made things even harder. Nothing is more difficult for a doctor than to tell a person he's afflicted with an illness for which there's no cure. The task is even more onerous when the illness destroys not only a person's body but his sanity as well.

Huntington's chorea—which afflicted folksinger Woody Guthrie—usually first shows up in middle age. At forty-three my patient is typical. The disease is caused by a single defective version of a gene lying on chromosome 4. What makes the illness particularly tragic is that approximately 50 percent of the children of people afflicted with Huntington's chorea will go on to develop Huntington's later in life. (Woody's son, singer Arlo Guthrie, is faced with this uncertainty.)

I had always believed that short of a cure for the illness, the next best thing would be a method of predicting which children would come down with Huntington's. On the basis of recent developments, however, I have changed my mind. Suffering psychological pain might well outweigh the gain of such knowledge.

At a meeting of the American Association for the Advancement of Science, a researcher, Michael Phelps, showed how biological abnormalities can be identified in the brains of patients with Huntington's chorea. He employed a PET scanner, which shows in motion-picture form the brain actually functioning, utilizing nutrients, performing chemical processes.

Phelps's main point was the PET scan can now show changes within the brain of a patient years before the illness manifests itself. "In 100 percent of the cases studied with PET," Phelps said, "we have pinpointed the altered chemical processes in the brains of the patients with symptoms even before they're detectable with other imaging procedures."

Over the ensuing six years, 50 percent of those patients with positive PET scans but no signs of the disease went on to develop Huntington's chorea. Within the next five years, depending on developments in the other 50 percent of the patients, neuroscientists will know for certain whether or not PET scans can provide a predictive test for Huntington's chorea.

For the sake of making a point, let's concede that the PET scanner is every bit as reliable as Phelps suggests. This translates into situations that I'm not sure I want to have any part of:

"I am sorry to inform you that my examination confirms Huntington's chorea. About 50 percent of your children are at risk for later coming down with the illness. If you wish, there is a test called a PET scan that can tell us for certain which of your children will get the disease."

Or:

"Your PET scan is typical of that of a patient with schizophrenia."

I want to emphasize that we're not talking about some science fiction fantasy. Not only will this test soon be available to any physician in the country, in all likelihood other diseases, too, will soon be diagnosed ahead of time by means of PET scans or other tests. As a result, physicians will be in the position of being able to tell people more than they may wish to know or, in many instances, could be expected to handle.

This situation can be expected to create a particularly intense conflict within those physicians for whom the need to cure, learn more about, or at least understand and "control" illnesses provides the greatest intellectual and emotional satisfaction.

This attitude is not restricted solely to the medical profession.

Our society at large is committed to the concept that "knowledge is power," that we are better off knowing than not knowing. We hate uncertainties, vagueness, having to "wait and see."

But in our urgency to know as much as we can about our present health and our health prospects, we may find ourselves facing situations wherein knowledge isn't helpful at all. Indeed, under certain circumstances it may be positively harmful.

For instance, if my mother or father suffered from manic depression and perhaps committed suicide, would I care to have myself hooked up to a device capable of telling me whether or not my scan pattern is "similar to" or "suggestive of" that of a person afflicted with a major mood disorder?

Speaking personally, almost certainly I would not. But do I have the right to decide about such a test for one of my patients, believing as I do that even to inform the patient of the existence of such a test is to create a conundrum that some individuals may be unprepared to deal with? In some individuals, such information might itself lead to a sense of hopelessness—even suicide. (Granted that with others such knowledge might serve as a spur toward getting treatment, repairing damaged relationships, getting the most out of the present moment, and so on.)

From a legal point of view, patients have a right to know everything the doctor knows about their condition. But just how aggressive should the physician be in his diagnostic endeavors? Although I have a clear legal obligation to "fully inform" my patient about all aspects of the present illness and how it may affect him or her, do I have an obligation to tell anything more? After all, I'm not being consulted as a seer or a prophet. It seems reasonable that I should confine my interventions to the illness at hand.

What about extending my efforts to other members of the patient's family who haven't sought my help directly? They may justifiably resent my intrusion into their lives. If my responsibility were to extend not just to my patient, but to my patient's children, where does this end? Public health measures—quarantine, vaccination programs—are only some of the areas in which the physician administers to a wider group than simply the individual who seeks his services. It will not be very long, I believe, before health programs will urge a similar widening of the physician's obligation to come up with extremely early diagnoses of diseases that ultimately will require long-term treatment or even institutional care.

Alzheimer's, schizophrenia, manic-depressive psychosis, obses- sive-compulsive disorders—these are now the principal candidates for predictive testing. Undoubtedly there will be more in the future. Notice, too, that all of the disorders mentioned affect behavior. This, in itself, creates an additional dilemma.

Learning that one may later suffer from depression or senility is a much different matter than learning about the likelihood of arthritis (another medical condition for which predictive tests based on genetics are in the offing). Throughout our lifetime we are taught to believe that "brain" and "body" mean something totally different from "mind" and "soul." To state that biological illnesses cause aberrant behavior, many people believe, places limitations on our free will that raise a serious question about our humanity: Are we any more than just the sum total of our bodies' flaws? New techniques such as PET scanners reinforce such re- evaluations.

Behavior is brain-based. Studying the brain helps us understand a host of dysfunctions. A dyslexia-caused reading problem, for instance, can be detected by studying a child's brain with a computer-enhanced electroencephalogram. Most intriguing is that in many instances these abnormalities can be detected even before the child is old enough to read.

While the early diagnosis of some disorders may be helpful and may even facilitate effective early intervention, many other disor- ders, including dyslexia, have so far frustrated our best attempts at treatment approaches that can be confidently anticipated to do any good.

Thus, whether the issue is a reading disability or a fatal illness, the puzzle remains the same: Should a patient be told about an illness that will not have much effect on the person for years to come, when, in the meantime, the knowledge can do little except cause worry and risk the patient's severe depression?

Such dilemmas are different from any faced in the past simply because technology, rather than providing a solution, as it has in the past (better drugs to better treat medical illnesses, refinements in surgical techniques, and so on), has itself become the problem.

As a result, future technological advances and refinements can be counted upon to intensify the often agonizing decision of who should know what and at what time. What tests should be ordered? By whom? Should tests that will only predict the appearance of the disease in the future be employed at all?

For now, I'm left with the dilemma of what to do with patients such as the one with Huntington's chorea. Certainly good and reasonable arguments can be made for the necessity of testing his children.

In a few years they may have potential spouses who reasonably might not wish to have babies with individuals who may end their days in madness after passing a flawed gene on to their offspring.

Insurance companies could certainly make use of information regarding a prospective applicant's chances of dying at an early age through an incurable disease. "Since your father died of this disease, before we write your policy, you must submit to a PET scan" could become a common requisite for being insured.

Illnesses may soon be diagnosable across generations, but these tests may reveal aspects of a person's emotional and intellectual life that he or she may have never suspected and might wish never to be informed about. Can a doctor be too candid? Can a patient's right to know be dangerous?

My patient with Huntington's chorea has three children who can be flown out to Los Angeles and, thanks to the wonders of modern technology, be hooked up to a PET scanner. Only one essential event must take place before that can happen, however. Somebody first has to tell my patient about the test and what it may portend.

Want to be let in on a secret? That person isn't going to be me.

o

A PROPER FORM
FOR EVERYTHING

My t'ai chi instructor emphasizes "form" in his teaching of this ancient Chinese martial art. Feet must be exactly shoulder width apart and no wider. Hands must move as if through water. Stiffness, rigidness, and clumsiness of any sort are greeted with horror.

One day while performing these relaxing but demanding exercises, I realized that there is a proper form for everything: fairly narrow parameters within which activities and structures must be accommodated lest chaos ensue.

Severe penalties are exacted for bad form in chess, tennis, and boxing. An inelegant chess move can lose the match. The tennis ball must be struck at just the right moment and with just the right amount of force, or the ball is lost in the net or perhaps missed altogether. If a punch is off target because of a slight lack of technique, a chance for a knockout has been missed. What's worse, it may have opened the way for a counterblow that could end the fight.

Form is also preeminent in the arts and determined by our biology, the way nature has constructed us. The time between beats is only between 0.63 seconds and 0.29 seconds in the range of tempos from adagio and andante to allegro and presto. If the cymbals come a fiftieth of a second too late, the audience winces. Form has been violated.

Carried to an extreme, form turns back on itself, becomes parody. The anorexic, believing that "thin is beautiful," goes too far, ends up a freak. Some weight lifters become so overdeveloped that their arms no longer move freely as they walk. The pursuit of the "perfect" form has led to the grotesque.

In biology good form is strictly and inexorably defined. Consider an animal's weight. Are there absolute limits to an animal's size, or could one exist weighing as much as one hundred tons? Bone artifacts from the dinosaur, the biggest land animal that ever lived, indicate that it may have weighed about eighty tons.

So why not a hundred-ton gargantuan? The answer is that the animal would require such a profound alteration of form, it could not survive. There are limits to the strength of bones and the power of muscles. Bone strength is proportional to cross-sectional area (a two-dimensional measure), whereas body weight is proportional to volume (a three-dimensional measure). Accordingly, the bone cross-sectional area must increase faster than body weight. Indeed, an animal weighing more than eighty tons would have to be composed *entirely* of bones frozen into immobility, because the creature's muscles would be unable to function. If the animal were to lie down—or, more likely, fall down of its own weight—its muscular system would be too weak to enable it to get up.

Form is also important to the human brain. As it turns out, just having a big brain is no guarantee of great intelligence. If it were, all six-foot-four men and women would be smarter than their five-foot-four counterparts. It's the brain-to-body ratio that's important, not brain size alone.

The size of the female pelvis imposes limitations on the brain's form. If the brain continued to expand, it would eventually get so big that the head couldn't pass through the birth canal. Nature has solved this problem of proper brain form in two ways. First, the greatest increase in brain size takes place *after* birth. Second, increased surface area is achieved without increasing brain volume by a process similar to what happens if you take a handkerchief and spread it out on a table, then roll it into a ball and put it into your pocket. The surface area remains the same, but the volume is greatly reduced. The same thing happens in the human brain. A fetus's hemispheres are smooth and unwrinkled. But an adult's looks like a gnarled walnut, because of billions of nerve cells sequestered deep below the surface. Just as in the handkerchief, a large surface area has been confined in a limited volume.

As the brain ages or is afflicted with disease, a person's walk, speech, and posture change. The form of the brain can be understood by those skilled in decoding such messages. But one does not have to be a neurologist to make such observations. Individuals who are clumsy, retarded, schizophrenic, or autistic; dancers; martial artists—often these people can be identified by the way they walk, which, basically, is form in motion.

On the whole, I think my t'ai chi teacher is right. The form must be exactly right. Excellence ultimately involves a preoccupation with form. Indeed, at the most basic level, structure, function, and form are inseparable. Or, as my t'ai chi teacher puts it: "After you do the form often enough, something marvelous happens: You and the form become one. Finally it begins to do you."

EMOTIONAL
STORMS

L ike most men, I get uncomfortable whenever other people, especially women, get emotional. Tears, raised voices, trembling, widely dilated pupils, frenetic gestures—these are the enemies of objectivity, or so most of us have been conditioned to believe. Furthermore, most of us would agree that, in general, rational people don't get emotional. Reason and emotionality are inversely related; don't get mad, get even. Such tenets imply that emotions and logical thought are distinctly different. We are conditioned to consider emotions as an inferior form of mental processing. We should be ashamed whenever we become "emotional."

Historically, scientific interest in emotions started with Darwin. His curiosity about them made him behave rather strangely to his own children, whom, we have it on good authority, he poked until they cried in order to study their facial expressions. In 1872 he published a book, *The Expression of the Emotions in Man and Animals*, containing these observations. It is still worth reading today. In it Darwin expressed his belief in the existence of specific fundamental emotions that occur in all people, wherever they may live, and whatever the conditions of their existence. Modern students of the emotions believe this, too. Indeed, emotions provide one of the great unifying themes in human biology.

But determining the *existence* of emotions is only part of the battle. Equally important are matters of *definition* (exactly what is an emotion?); *origin* (what causes emotions?); and *individuality* (why are some people so much more susceptible to emotions than others?).

To take up the last question first, a psychiatrist in Florence, Italy, Graziella Magherini, has observed that some people encountering a great work of art in one of Florence's museums undergo an intense "storm of emotions." They may faint; become ecstatic; experience a rapid acceleration of heart rate or disorientation, or even delusions of omnipotence or grandiosity. "An evocative painting or statue can produce unpredictable results," Magherini says. Not every visitor to the museum is susceptible to such emotional storms. Usually they affect only those with histories of nervous disorders, the fatigued, those traveling alone, the overly impressionable. In these instances of the Stendhal syndrome—named after the nineteenth-century French writer who experienced something similar while gazing at the frescoes in the Church of Santa Croce—it's clear that emotions are tightly linked with meaning. In other words, for every sufferer from the Stendhal syndrome, there are undoubtedly dozens of distinctly unemotional tourists who are bored and can't wait to get out of the museum and head for the nearest bar.

Concerning the origin of emotions, William James came up with a theory in 1884 that, if the phrase had been current at the time, would have been described as completely "off the wall." James held that our visceral reactions—the racing heart, the sweating, the hollow feeling in the pit of the stomach, and so on—constitute the origin of our emotions.

"Our feelings of (bodily) changes as they occur is the emotion," as James put it. In short, "We feel sorry because we cry . . . not that we cry because we are sorry."

James believed that bodily changes follow in the wake of some exciting event and that the perception of these changes constitutes the emotion. The Danish physician Carl Lange independently proposed something similar, but with a slightly different emphasis. He contended that emotions are localized in the vasomotor system, which controls the contraction of our blood vessels. When the system is stimulated, said Lange, emotions are experienced.

"We owe all the emotional side of our mental life, our joys and sorrows, our happy and unhappy hours, to our vasomotor system," writes Lange. "If the impressions which fall upon our senses did not possess the power of stimulating it, we would wander through life unsympathetic and passionless, all impressions of the outer world would only enrich our experience, increase our knowledge, but would arouse neither joy nor anger, would give us neither care nor fear."

The so-called James/Lange theory of emotions came in for a lot of criticism in the 1920s. The physiologist Walter Cannon made the point that emotions still exist even when the brain is separated from visceral organs. In support of his premise, Cannon cited the case of Dana, a forty-year-old woman who broke her neck in a fall from a horse. Despite her total paralysis and anesthesia from the neck down, she continued to experience and express the normal range of emotions. Cannon had three additional criticisms. First, emotions don't seem to differ very much when it comes to bodily responses (i.e., the heart rate can accelerate from pleasurable anticipation or fear). Second, heart rate and change in breathing patterns occur relatively slowly, whereas emotions arise seemingly instantaneously. Finally, not everyone experiences the same emotions when internal bodily states are deliberately induced by drugs. A stimulant that accelerates the sympathetic nervous system may induce anxiety in some people and no particular emotion at all in others. When it comes to the origin of emotions, context is more important than explanations based on physiology.

As with the art gallery experience in Florence, emotions depend on meaning. Variables such as expectations, preconceptions, the degree of control one maintains and experiences when undergoing something new and unfamiliar can make the difference between equanimity and pure terror. For instance, I've noted that patients undergoing an MRI examination experience different emotions according to how well they are prepared for the test. During the test the patient, after lying down on a moving table, is enclosed in a drumlike space with only a few inches separating the tip of his nose from the top of the cylinder. Speaking both personally and professionally, I can say that undergoing an MRI can be a horribly claustrophobic experience or only a mildly unpleasant one, depending on what one has been told beforehand about the test. In almost all patients the heart rate increases, the breathing pattern alters, and restlessness ensues. One patient, not knowing what to expect, experiences acute panic. But another patient, forewarned and thereby emotionally forearmed, closes his eyes, ignores the heart rate and breathing changes, and remains calm.

Despite our tendency to think otherwise, emotions cannot be neatly walled off from rationality like a doddering uncle confined to an attic room. Nor are emotions just remnants of our prehistoric past, heirlooms of those of our forefathers who swung from trees. Instead, emotions arise in response to change, failures of habitual response patterns, failed expectations, almost anything that requires searching for an explanation for the new and unexpected.

"The human world is full of emotions, not because we are animals at heart, but rather because it is still full of signals that elate or threaten, and replete with events and people that produce discrepancies and interruptions," writes psychologist George Mandler, author of *Mind and Body*.

Answering the most knotty question of all—What is an emotion?—is difficult because modern science often doesn't provide very satisfying answers to questions like this. It's better at definitions such as those already discussed. But exploring meanings isn't very helpful when it comes to emotions, with all of their subtlety. Defining an emotion is like trying to capture the smile of the Cheshire cat.

As an illustration of my point, consider this question: Are you an anxious person? You may answer, in perfect honesty, no. Yet measurements of anxiety involving your heart rate, pupillary dilatation, and sympathetic arousal may indicate otherwise. In such a situation the subjective frame of your answer ("No, I'm not anxious") is in direct contradiction to objective measurements of your anxiety.

So are you anxious or are you not? Harvard psychologist Jerome Kagan suggests that such a question is not only unanswerable, but no longer even meaningful at the level of a yes or no response. Anxiety, along with other emotions, such as love, hate, longing— select any emotion about which you are curious—is neither easily defined nor something everyone can agree about. In fact, anxiety, along with other emotions, is, in Kagan's words, an "unstable idea." It varies greatly according to the dictates of the period, the social situation, the interests and prejudices of the investigator, and, finally, the techniques and technologies employed to investigate anxiety.

Physiological variables and our subjective state are pretty much in accord in most of us most of the time. But every day in my neuropsychiatric practice I treat people whose thoughts, emotions, and physiological processes are out of sync. Free-floating anxiety, for example, makes one person feel vaguely threatened and uneasy. His heart rate, blood pressure, muscle tension, and breathing patterns reflect a deep-seated unease, yet the patient has no idea why he feels anxious. He begs me for an explanation; he hopes against hope that there is some reason that can be identified and ultimately addressed.

A similar split between thought and feelings can be observed in patients given to panic attacks. These usually retiring and somewhat depressed individuals function normally until, with the suddenness of a lightning bolt, they are hit by a dreaded attack. Feelings of dissolution, fears of imminent death, the sensation of strangling, the horror of entering into a psychic black hole—these are the emotions brought on by a panic attack.

For both those who are prone to anxiety and those given to panic attacks, bodily changes such as an accelerating heart rate are interpreted as foreshadowing something awful. In response such individuals construct scenarios capable of explaining the depth and intensity of these agonizing emotions. Finally, after the anxiety has subsided, they establish rituals in order to avoid re-creating the situation that caused the anxiety attack. Agoraphobia, which in Greek means fear of the marketplace, probably originated as a description of one anxious person who dealt with his anxiety in the marketplace by avoiding return trips there.

As an explanation for discrepancies between thinking and emotion I favor the view—certainly not original with me—that these different aspects of mind result from activity generated at different levels of the brain. On occasion a component of this dynamic system can break out into an autonomous rhythm of its own, like a rebellious teenager who storms out of the house and frets away the rest of the evening at an emotional tempo different from other family members'.

Studies of split brain patients make a similar point. After communication links between hemispheres are sectioned, feelings of embarrassment, dismay, or even amusement can be induced without a patient's even knowing why. Recall that when an experimenter projected a picture of a naked person to the right hemisphere, the split brain patient became embarrassed and didn't know why. That dissociation between knowledge and emotion was the result of the surgical disconnection of the right hemisphere from the left hemisphere, which is responsible for language. But even though these perceptions can't be verbally described, they can still induce appropriate emotions.

Take another example: In schizophrenics, the personality "split" is not one of multiple selves, a common misconception. Rather, it is a schism between thinking and feeling. Tales of dreadful woe may be recounted by a schizophrenic in a tone of laughter or banter. Tears instead of laughter may be evoked when a schizophrenic hears a joke. At all times the mood or affect is inappropriate to the situation discussed. Once again, the emotions of that rebellious teenager are rocking and rolling to a rhythm all their own.

Happily for us, the rhythms of our thought and emotions usually interact with the grace and responsiveness of two perfectly trained dancers. That's why I'm uncomfortable around people whose thoughts and emotions are out of sync or who too readily display negative emotions and feelings such as anger for having suffered some unnamed injustice. Why do I react with such acute discomfort? Because those individuals, feeling bad, are demanding something of me that I hope to provide but cannot always be certain that I do. And I want to respond compassionately to the one plea from another human being that a doctor should never ignore. See how I suffer. . . . You can help me. . . . *Please* do.

And of course I do try. And sometimes my knowledge about the ways that emotions and thought diverge allows me to succeed.

o

LUCID DREAMING ON DEMAND

At a conference on the brain I spoke with coparticipant Stephen LaBerge, a research associate at Stanford University and possibly the world's most accomplished practitioner of the art of lucid dreaming. "What's lucid dreaming?" you ask. Well, if you're dreaming, and aware that you're dreaming, then you're having a lucid dream. The advantage of a lucid dream is that you can enter the dream, change its script, introduce new characters, and engage in heroic exploits beyond your most extravagant Walter Mitty fantasies.

LaBerge claims that after some instruction and practice, we all can learn to enter our dreams. After additional practice we may even become accomplished "oneironauts." (*Oneiros* is Greek for dream.)

As an aid toward achieving proficiency in lucid dreaming, La-Berge has developed "lucid dream induction goggles," modified swim goggles that flash a soft red light whenever the subject enters the REM (rapid eye movement) state, within which all dream activity takes place. The light reminds the sleeper that he or she is asleep and that anything happening at the moment is likely to be a dream.

A less high-tech approach to dreams was suggested to me a few weeks later by J. Allen Hobson, researcher at the Harvard University Dream Laboratory and author of *The Dreaming Brain*. "The presleep command 'I will remember my dreams,' repeated nightly, was usually adequate to produce dramatically increased dream recall within three to five weeks of placing a dream journal at one's bedside," Hobson told me.

After personally trying Hobson's method, I can attest that it works.

But is there any advantage to remembering past dreams or entering into present ones? Are dreams really meaningful?

The psychoanalyst's interpretation of dream symbols, Freud claimed, could put the patient in touch with his unconscious. Since the unconscious appears within dreams in a disguised form (the latent content) by means of symbols standing in for anxiety-provoking subjects (usually violence or sexuality), psychoanalysts hold that the dreamer has little chance of understanding his dreams. Instead, the dreams have to be interpreted by the analyst.

Hobson now challenges this precept by suggesting the breathtakingly audacious idea that there is no latent content to dreams; rather, dreams mean exactly what they seem to mean. "I think that most dreams are neither obscure nor bowdlerized, but rather transparent and unedited. They contain clearly meaningful, undisguised, highly conflictual impulses worthy of note by the dreamer (and any interpretative assistant)."

Freud and Hobson agree that dreams are meaningful; they differ only on the degree of a dream's transparency. But if dreams are so meaningful, why is it that we recall so few of them? Surely from the evolutionary point of view a process capable of conveying insights, novel interpretations, and the solution to problems—and dreams can provide all of these—should be readily available and accessible to the dreamer upon awakening.

One of the reasons that dreams are not so accessible is that not everybody can handle the intensely emotional, illogical content and organization that characterize dreams. In a sense a dream is a temporary psychosis. "All of the major signs of mental illness can be imitated by normal minds in the normal state of dreaming," writes Hobson in *The Dreaming Brain*. "The study of dreams is a study of a model of mental illness."

But whatever the dream and however unusual or disturbing its content, the dreamer, once awakened, faces an important decision: how much credence to give to something that occurred in a dream.

The classic Greek author Artemidorus held that dreams are prophetic, and that by analyzing your dreams, you could know your future. Few people other than the extremely superstitious hold to this view now. But, on the other hand, I would suggest that if you completely ignore your dreams, you do so at your own peril.

For instance, what would you do if you had three dreams over a week or so in which you were killed or seriously injured in your sports car? Probably nothing. But suppose that in that period you were involved in a minor accident and then a near collision at a speed that would have guaranteed a not-so-minor result? Would you wait for the third event? Or would you do as I did and sell the car?

Such dreams are explained, I believe, as a subconscious expression of one's own, or someone else's, intuition or hunch. "If you keep driving so fast, you're going to get into an accident," my wife had been telling me for several weeks prior to the dream. No problem in explaining those accident dreams.

But there are other examples where the influence of intuitions and hunches is more opaque. What does one make of a dream in which a casual acquaintance appears and tells you that a good friend or lover is a "dangerous person" and not to be trusted? Would *you* break off the relationship? That depends, I suspect, on whether you are comfortable in the situation in the first place. Dreams provide grand excuses for doing or not doing what you have already decided should or should not be done.

All of which makes Stephen LaBerge's invitation to become a lucid dreamer more interesting and inviting. Imagine being able to enter the dream, slow down the car, and avoid the accident. Or ask why the person holds such negative feelings about your friend or lover.

Most appealing of all would be the cocktail party possibilities. Wouldn't it be fun to tell someone that, in addition to all of the other things you do, you're an accomplished oneironaut?

o

MIND
MURDER

He's trying to murder my mind," she said. Then she began to cry softly.

At the time, a decade ago, I wasn't certain what my thirty-two-year-old patient meant by her description of her husband's behavior. Nothing she had told me about him seemed to justify a word like *murder*. And what exactly did she mean by "mind murder"? Her explanation at the time went something like this: "My husband says one thing, but I can tell by his tone of voice that he means just the opposite."

I wrote in my notebook, "Two messages seem to be involved in mind murder. One is explicit and says one thing. The second message is subliminal, conveyed primarily by tone, and negates the first."

In the intervening years I've been on the alert for mind murder, and I've found it all around me.

• An eight-year-old girl: "Mommy, why can't I go to the movies with the other kids? You're so mean sometimes!"

Mother: "Now, that's not a nice thing to say to your mother. I've only got your best interests at heart. You know that I love you." But the word *love* in the last sentence comes out sounding as if the girl's mother had said *hate*.

• "You married men get everything you want. But I know one thing you're not going to get," says the lovely young woman as she crosses and uncrosses her recently waxed legs. "I've got your family's interests at heart. I don't want things to get out of control."

The child wants to believe her mother loves her, but the tone, for reasons she can't explain, makes her uneasy and nervous. The married man finds himself reminded of his family obligations at the moment those lovely legs are arousing his lust.

Another example from a rather seriously disturbed patient. "You should have the Congressional Medal of Spit," a schizophrenic woman said to her psychiatrist, who wrote in his notes, "The first seven words of that eight-word sentence conveyed heartfelt admiration, but the last one, said with no break at all in the rhythm of her speech, was uttered in unalloyed contempt."

"How glad I am to see you" can be an expression of genuine joy or sarcasm, depending on the inflection of the word *glad*. Comedians often achieve their effects by deliberately creating a dissonance between what's said and the manner in which it's said.

Perhaps an old joke defines mind murder best: What did the sadist do to the masochist? Answer: Nothing.

In recent years neuroscientists have made discoveries about the brain that have shed light on the dynamics of mind murder. The brain's right hemisphere, we now know, is important for providing emotional tone and timbre.

Certain patients with brain injury in their right hemisphere can't generate the emotional state appropriate to what they say. Others can generate their own appropriate emotions but can't respond properly to the emotional ambiences of other people's words. "You're a real genius" convinces them that the speaker is flattering their intelligence, but they remain unaware that the contemptuous way *genius* was said implies, instead, something like nitwit.

Communication depends only partially on the words that are said. Equally important are the ways things are said, thus making possible irony, humor, flattery, admiration, and other subtleties of expression. Such subtleties also provide psychological sadists with a method for murdering another person's mind. Remember that old movie *Gaslight*? The title has been turned into a verb. If you want to "gaslight" somebody, you wait until he or she says something mildly controversial in front of other people and then you do things like raise your eyebrows, roll your eyes, or make sudden gestures of embarrassment. You can suggest, without saying a word, that your intended victim is, well, unstable, not at all reliable. Milder forms of the same technique can be used for social purposes.

"We'd love to have you visit," I said two days ago to a person who, if he had visited me here on Martha's Vineyard, would have so skewed my writing schedule that the essay you're now reading would never have been written. Earlier in the evening I had practiced inflecting the word *love* so that the disparity between message and delivery would be obvious enough to be effective but not so obvious as to offend.

How do I justify doing what I have just so clearly criticized in others? Simple. I think it makes a good deal of difference whether word-emotional dissonances are deliberately created with full knowledge of what's going on or whether they occur outside the conscious intent of the speaker. It also is important that mind murder not be deliberately used for destructive means. But even making that distinction isn't always easy. In fact, that is a problem with mind murder. Often the perpetrator cannot be confronted because the processes are occurring outside his awareness. But in instances involving conscious intent, such as my lukewarm invitation, communication is still possible if a listener is perceptive enough: "Listen, Richard . . . you don't sound very excited about my coming. If you don't want me to visit, then just say so and let's dispense with the games." "Okay, Roger. If you want it straight, please don't come to visit; I've got too many things to do."

Mind murder exists because some people have a need to try to make life simpler than it usually is. The mother mentioned in this essay loves her child in her own way but resents the child's restrictions on her freedom. Her brain can't seem to process this conflict, so she chooses to express only one side of it by a subliminally hostile tone of voice, thus murdering her child's mind. And the lovely young lady with the sensational legs would surely give her married friend what she thinks he wants if only the circumstances were different (or so she says).

I, too, am now a victim of mind murder. When she finished reading what you've just finished reading, my wife smiled and said: "The piece is interesting, but you're not really serious about this mind murder stuff, now, are you?"

THE TWO REALITIES
OF THE MIND

A neurology professor once taught me something very important about science. He insisted that "one must not only try to be right, but be right for the right reasons."

By this he meant that it isn't enough merely to diagnose a condition correctly. The physician also has to justify in painstaking detail that only one diagnosis is correct.

I understood the subtle meaning of his requirement on the morning when I expounded at great length and to my professor's complete satisfaction a diagnosis that, it turned out, he knew at the time was wrong. He let me continue, he said later, because "at this point in your training it's more important that you went about it correctly. This time you were wrong. The next time you may be right for the right reasons."

History is filled with thinkers and scientists who have employed the right and wrong reasons with varying results. Often they have been correct in their conclusions. But equally often, as with my diagnosis, they've turned out to have been mistaken. Sometimes it may not even be possible to be certain whether the right reasons are going to lead to the right conclusions.

For instance, Plato decided that the brain was the organ of the soul or the mind. He based his reasoning on the belief that the sphere was the "perfect geometric shape." The head is nearly spherical and therefore, Plato concluded, must be the container for the physical embodiment of man's spiritual essence. The reasoning is impeccable, but few of us would concede that the supposed perfection of the sphere provides an adequate basis for his choice of the brain. In short, most of us would agree that Plato was right for the wrong reasons.

Aristotle went about things a bit differently. Observing that a living body is warm and a dead one cold, he sought the source of this warmth: the blood. Because the heart, not the brain, pumps the blood, he reasoned, the heart has to originate the warmth and be the site of the soul. Aristotle was wrong, but for reasons that would have pleased my professor: the employment of a logical argument (the right reasons) based on a rudimentary form of experimentation.

Because of the value we place on modern science, we laud Aristotle, the originator of the scientific method, as a genius. Plato, by contrast, is considered by most scientists a mystic noted for his insistence that the senses are unreliable.

But I prefer to think of the difference between Plato and Aristotle in another way. Both employed the "right reasons," but they were dealing with two separate and distinct levels of reality: the objective and the subjective. Plato and Aristotle differed essentially over their estimation of the importance of subjectivity.

To appreciate the significance of these differences, consider where Aristotle's scientific method led in regard to the nature of the mind. Thoughts or moments of conscious awareness cannot be detected by sight, sound, or taste. All of us regularly experience them, but they cannot be demonstrated to the satisfaction of the scientist. For the longest time, therefore, they were ignored by behaviorists and others who insisted that science should concern itself with only objectively verifiable reality.

Plato and his followers, meanwhile, insisted on the importance of inner experience. They believed that we aren't simply conditioned by our environments, but we react and respond to them. "I think, therefore I am" is how Descartes described the process. To someone in touch with his inner experience, this aphorism could be modified to "I am, therefore I think." In other words, inner experience is as important as anything that can be established by modern science.

Modern brain research has developed an instrument proving that Plato was right. Our inner experience can, in fact, be demonstrated with scientific objectivity. The technique, known as positron emission tomography, or PET, involves the injection of a radioactively tagged isotope into a vein. The molecule eventually enters the brain, especially those brain cells most active at a given time. The accumulated isotope produces a color-coded map of brain activity.

Some truly astounding things have been learned about the inner landscapes of our mind in the short time that PET scanning has been available. Someone looking at a white light yields one PET scan image. Sitting on the campus of UCLA on a summer afternoon results in a more dramatically vivid image. A musician listening to music displays a different color-coded image than a listener with no musical training. In other experiments the PET scan changes in response to different kinds of mental activity.

PET scans make it possible to study the internal functioning of the brain. Certain forms of mental illness, such as schizophrenia and manic depression, are accompanied by specific PET scan patterns, or signatures. But what is most exciting is that for the first time in history, inner experiences can be demonstrated by PET scanning in a way that conforms to the objectivity requirements of scientists, confirming that reality has both objective and subjective components. Here in the Western world we have emphasized objective observable phenomena to the exclusion of inner experience. Thinkers in the Eastern tradition have always insisted on the validity of inner experience. Now, thanks to PET scans, these two views can be reconciled.

Reconsidering the two-thousand-year-old debate between Aristotle and Plato, I realize that both of these intellectual giants were right, and for the right reasons. Scientific experimentation and observation are vital in learning about the outer, objective world. But we should not ignore what we think, how we feel, our own intuitions. To do so is to deny a huge and essential aspect of reality: the inner landscape of our own minds.

o

THE LAST
GRADE OF MASTERY

"I know but one freedom and that is the
freedom of the mind."

ANTOINE DE SAINT EXUPÉRY.

reud once remarked that hysterics suffer from reminis-
cences. Unresolved events from the past, symbolically
rearranged in the unconscious by repressive forces, burst
forth in a series of psychologically rather than physically
caused symptoms—i.e., "hysterical" paralysis, blindness, and so
on.

With equal justification Freud could have claimed that all people afflicted with emotional disturbances suffer as a result of the
contents of their own minds. With obsessives, the suffering comes
as a result of things that can't be suppressed but keep coming back
to torture and agitate the sufferer. Depressives relive the past as a
series of paths not taken and opportunities missed. The anxious
man or woman has a foreboding of dangerous or unpleasant events
that are always about to happen. And for the victims of posttrau-
matic stress disorder, with its nightmares and flashbacks of horrific
experiences, life becomes a series of replays of events that the
sufferer wishes desperately to forget.

But suffering due to the contents of one's own mind is not by any
means restricted to instances of emotional illness. Every one of us
has a favorite list of topics we don't want to think about. Studies of
"unwanted thoughts" reported by college students revealed (in
order of more to less frequency) problems with relationships (jealousy, being rejected, loneliness, difficulties in getting along with

others); school concerns (failure, not completing assignments on time); general worries about the past and future; the death of loved ones and friends; fear of being victimized (rape, robbery); money failures; worries about physical appearance; sexual problems; health concerns regarding food and eating.

Unwanted thoughts teach us that the more we attempt to manage the mind's contents, control the things that we think about, the more we become ensnared in what we're trying *not* to think about. Several experiments have made this point, the most famous conducted by Daniel M. Wegner, chairman of the psychology department at Trinity University in San Antonio, Texas.

Wegner's experiments duplicated in a more scientifically rigorous fashion a thought experiment first suggested by the novelist Fyodor Dostoevsky: "Try not to think about a white bear," Wegner and his associates told their subjects. Despite the subjects' best efforts, however, the white bear kept reappearing in their thoughts and spontaneous statements. (They had been instructed to say aloud everything that came to mind.) Over a five-minute period the white bear was mentioned between six and fifteen times!

Such findings may surprise you, even shock you. After all, if you can't control what enters your own mind, then what can you control? Indeed, it's this attitude ("Even though I can't control things in the external world around me, I can certainly control my own inner world. . . . After all, that's me!") that creates anguish when a person's inner world is experienced as unpredictable and, what's worse, uncontrollable.

But why can't we successfully suppress thoughts that we don't want?

To answer this question, let your attention wander just a bit to some of the things that are occurring around you as you're reading. In my case, a dog is barking in the yard next door, an airplane is flying overhead, a jogger is about halfway across my line of sight along the road in front of my window. All of these vaguely formulated impressions and thoughts are occurring all at once; none is more pressing than the other. They form a background to the process occupying me at the moment, i.e., writing this essay.

Now imagine that I allow or perhaps purposely select one of these thoughts to occupy center stage in the theater of my consciousness. Let's say at a certain moment the barking of the dog next door becomes so annoying that I can't think of anything else and can no longer write. What is more, try as I might, I can't get the dog's barking off my mind. In desperation I encourage myself to concentrate harder, ignore the barking, stop thinking about the dog. At this point my consciousness is trapped in a paradox: the dog's barking and my attempts to ignore the barking occur simultaneously in my consciousness. The self-instruction "stop thinking of the dog's barking" exists as a metathought: an instruction for the conscious mind to change its own contents. As Wegner puts it in his book *White Bears and Other Unwanted Thoughts*, the "suppression metathought ('I'd rather not think of a white bear') is here, but the thought ('white bear') is here, too. As long as we continue to hold the metathought in the conscious window the thought will be there, too. Current consciousness is unable to think itself out of having a thought because this entails thinking the thought."

Attempts to prevail in this struggle to banish forever an unwanted thought intensify one's mental anguish and suffering. If additional efforts are made, the deadlock between the thought and the attempt to banish the thought may lead to forms of mental illness. Severe obsessions, depressions, or psychotic reactions marked by panic, disorganization, and the conviction that one is losing one's mind are just a few of the terrifying possibilities.

Always we encounter this paradox about the human mind: when it comes to mental control, the harder one tries, the worse things get. But this paradox is not limited to unwanted thoughts. Too intense a desire for getting to sleep can almost be guaranteed to result in a night of sleepless tossing and turning. Too much determination to be sexually successful leads not to enhanced performance, but to impotence, frigidity, inhibitions of sexual desire, and other dysfunctions. Each of these instances describes a mind locked in a struggle between its contents and the independent but competing wish to alter those contents.

But acceptance of our unwanted thoughts deprives them of their capacity to make us suffer. Wegner put it with charming simplicity: "Once we stop suppressing, by definition, we no longer have thoughts we do not want." Entertaining rather than banishing uncomfortable or disturbing thoughts is the surest way of achieving perhaps one of our most important freedoms.

How ironic that the rule for mental control involves the least controlling intellectual and emotional attitudes: let go, forget yourself, lighten up . . . you're not the only one in the world who has thoughts he doesn't want to think.

If we can learn to inwardly embrace these attitudes, then there's hope that we can even achieve what the Master in *Zen in the Art of Archery* proclaims as the "last grade of mastery."

> *"You worry yourself unnecessarily," the Master comforted me. "Put the thought of hitting right out of your mind! You can be a Master even if every shot does not hit. The hits on the target are only the outward proof and confirmation of your purposelessness at its highest, of your egolessness, your self-abandonment or whatever you like to call this state. There are different grades of mastery, and only when you've made the last grade will you be sure of not missing the goal."*

o

NOBODY AT HOME

I magine a household of people with different physical limitations. Some cannot see; some are deaf; some cannot speak; some have no memory; still others are paralyzed. But by improving various patterns of cooperation, they discover that they can get along. No single individual, however, seems to orchestrate the cooperation. The household lacks a leader.

Someone unacquainted with the occupants of this strange household would find it difficult to figure out the group's organizational structure. It would be even harder (and counterintuitive as well) to understand how the occupants can perform as a group in ways that no single one of them can perform on his own. It would violate our understanding of how the world works to imagine that actions requiring fairly sophisticated processing (timely payment of bills, answering letters, and so on) could take place in the absence of some kind of hierarchy. We would assume that in order for the household to function, some person or group of persons (or perhaps all of the occupants of the household as a group) must set down rules about what should be done, when, and by whom.

Consider this household as a possible metaphor for the human brain, and an important question arises immediately: Is this really how the brain works? The fairest answer is yes and no. In some ways the brain is organized like the household of the blind, the lame, and the forgetful. But in other ways the brain shows signs of a hierarchy.

Let's take the hierarchical arrangement first. To do so it is necessary to have some slight acquaintance with John Hughlings Jackson, a bearded and introverted neurologist born in 1835. Hughlings Jackson, as he preferred to be known, was definitely not a party animal. He was reclusive. In the quiet of his study he pondered a lot and read philosophy, particularly the works of Herbert Spencer.

It was Spencer, not Darwin, who coined the phrase "survival of the fittest." But Spencer's definition of that term was different from Darwin's. Spencer did not think of evolution as a hit-or-miss affair in which species successfully adapted themselves to their environments by chance genetic mutation. Instead, he was an expansive, enthusiastic advocate of progress, a believer in the notion that things always get better and better. He believed in a straight progression from the simple to the complex, from the mundane to the divine.

Spencer's vision of a hierarchical society with "primitive" lower orders kept in their proper place by more sophisticated upper orders appealed to Hughlings Jackson, a temperate, conservative man whose silences and laconic utterances sometimes rivaled those of the speechless patients who regularly came under his care. But to be fair to Hughlings Jackson, he was very much a product of his age. To a generation still haunted by memories of the French Revolution, a hierarchical social organization made a great deal of sense. If the higher order lessened its control, anarchy would be unleashed.

By studying the human brain, Hughlings Jackson found much to justify his concept of hierarchical organization. For every brain function—speech, movement, sensation, consciousness, and so on—Jackson perceived a hierarchy of three levels, each of which exerted control over the level below. If the structure in a higher level was rendered inactive by, say, a stroke or a tumor, the function of a lower level, normally held in check, was released with the fury of a revolutionary storming a barricade. For instance, a stroke involving the language center may be followed by episodes of crying, agitation, and frustrated attempts to communicate by gesture. To Hughlings Jackson "control" and "release" were the terms that explained such developments. Evolution added progressively higher levels of control both in the species and in the individual. The opposite process, dissolution, led to a loss of higher cortical levels, both in the brain and in the larger social order. (The French social psychologist Gustav LeBon adapted Hughlings Jackson's neurologic hierarchy and applied it to the study of people in crowds. A mob, according to LeBon, corresponded to a "spinal man," an organism powered only by reflex and completely cut off from the temporizing influence of reason and judgment.)

Although Hughlings Jackson never carried out an experiment in his life—favoring instead the study of natural experiments carried out on the brain by nature—he hit upon a theory of brain organization that has a lot to recommend it.

The brain seems to be organized along lines compatible with Hughlings Jackson's thinking. It can be divided into three gross sections. The forebrain, the topmost level, mediates conscious awareness, intention, and personality. The midbrain processes automatic activities, such as walking, which operate quite satisfactorily without conscious interference. And the hindbrain, or brain stem, contains centers for the regulation of such fundamental activities as breathing and control of heart rate, temperature, and the circulation of the blood. Breakdowns of the brain's higher structures (the forebrain) result in deficiencies and ineptitudes in functioning (loss of speech or abstract thought) that the "mob" down below, at the levels of the midbrain and hindbrain, cannot compensate for.

For instance, a person afflicted with Alzheimer's disease loses his memory before losing the capacity to feed himself. He relinquishes his interest in Mozart prior to the time he stops reading the newspaper. Sophisticated skills such as bridge or chess deteriorate before the patient loses the knowledge of how to go about retrieving a phone number from the information operator.

Other instances of normal and not-so-normal brain processing don't fit into Hughlings Jackson's conception of a hierarchy. These exceptions are more consistent with the strange household of people mentioned at the beginning of this essay, which functions without a leader by simply letting everyone do what he does best.

For instance, techniques have been developed for recording the activity of single nerve cells. Two Harvard University neuroscientists, David Hubel and Torsten Wiesel, shared the Nobel Prize for their location of cells in the visual cortex that respond to increasingly complex features of the world—a spot of light, a bar, a moving bar, and so on. Moreover, different areas specialize in the analysis of particular visual features. Cells in one area are sensitive to the orientation of simple lines and edges. Cells in another area respond to wavelengths; still others to movement. In essence, all of the elements are present for a hierarchy such as Hughlings Jackson proposed, extending from the simple to the complex.

But additional studies of the visual cortex suggest that the arrangement may be less hierarchical. Indeed, it may function quite satisfactorily without the need for a "pecking order" wherein one cell "controls" the functional relations of cells subservient to it.

If one traces the communications of one visual area to another, as has been done by a researcher at the University College, London, one discovers that the relationships of the different visual areas to one another do not follow a linear or hierarchical arrangement. Rather, these layers form a highly distributed processing system. One area, in addition to analyzing lines and edges, assembles information about different aspects of the visual world, such as motion and contrast. The mechanics of how all this visual information is recombined remains a tantalizing but as yet unsolved mystery.

Rather than one fairly restricted visual area in the brain, there are actually many smaller regions that operate in a modular fashion, with the respective modules remaining as independent as possible from each other. Once visual information is encoded within the brain, it is widely distributed, entering into networks where it is associated with information from many other sources.

The hypothalamus, for instance, contains cells that respond to the sight of food, but that do so only when the animal is hungry. Certain brain cells located in the lower regions of the temporal lobes respond selectively to faces. "Seeing," in other words, exists always within a context, is not precisely localizable. Most notably, it always involves networks of cells acting in concert.

But how does such a system make possible a coherent experience of the world? If the brain operates in a modular manner (each area functioning relatively independent of every other and processing a separate aspect of reality), who or what brings about the ultimate synthesis? As far as anyone can tell at this point, the brain has no "center" responsible for analyzing and reconstructing into a simple, meaningful whole all the information entering it. This is a situation similar to that of the household operating with mutual cooperation: each person doing what he does best, rather than a hierarchical arrangement starting with a leader and working downward. Organization exists; principles of organization can be discovered. But there appears to be no "organizer."

For the longest time I found this lack of an organizer within the brain extremely disturbing. It affronted my autonomy, my sense of myself as a unity in charge of my fate. I looked for some way to reconcile my subjective sense of myself as unified with the neurological findings that suggest that I'm more like a confederacy. Two insights occurred to me.

First, metaphors are always borrowed from current social and political situations. It is foolish therefore to consider any metaphor for the brain as definitive. Changes in the social and political worlds will present changes in the metaphors we employ to understand the brain. Thus our search for an organizer within the brain may be nothing more than a metaphor from earlier, simpler times marked by social and political hierarchies of dominance, control, and command.

Second, our insistence that our mental landscape is a unified one coincides for most of us with a belief that our relationship to the rest of the world is not unified. According to this way of thinking, the world "out there" is like a movie, and we are the viewers of the movie. Yet philosophers, particularly those from the East, have always insisted on the unity of ourselves and the world. But how can we be one with the world when we experience ourselves as separate? Zen master Dainin Katagiri suggested a solution of this puzzle to me. He did so by way of the following thought experiment.

Let us imagine you are climbing up a mountain cliff. That situation is just like being on the verge of life and death. There is no way to escape; you cannot complain. If you are there, all you have to do is just be there. If you act instinctively, you could die. If you are nervous, you could die. Should you depend on the intellect, you could also die. So you have to depend on the mountain, your mind, and all the circumstances. You have to watch carefully and understand. Your consciousness must be clear and know what is going on there. Then, after using your best understanding, your body and mind should depend on just one step. This is action. This is the process of one step without being nervous about what will happen in the next moment, or thinking about when you will reach the peak, or how far down the bottom is, or who is climbing, or how much farther you can keep going like this, or that you could die. There is nothing to think about, nothing to depend on. All that we have to do is just be there using all the things we already have: consciousness, mind, mountain, and the weather. Then we have to act. Just take one step, a pretty simple step.

What is this one step? Is it to understand about living by studying about philosophy or psychology? I don't think so. Finally they must be thrown away. All we have to do is just live. Take one step, and that step must be stable. This means that after using your consciousness with your best effort, then act, wholeheartedly. This one step is really not just one step; it is the universe, including the mountains, your mind, and your consciousness. All things are completely melted into one step. What is one step? One step is the mountain. One step is the weather. One step is you. One step is the true way to live. It is really to attain the Way.

In Katagiri's image the mountain and the weather and the contents of the climber's mind form a unity. Yet at the same time each element retains its separate identity. Depending on circumstances, one or the other may determine whether the climber reaches the top of the mountain or plunges to his death. Hierarchical arrangements are of little importance here. Or in the brain. The brain's organization lacks both a central organizer and a hierarchical chain of command.

What would be a suitable metaphor for such an arrangement? My thoughts return to the strange household mentioned at the beginning of this essay. So many people performing their limited activities quite satisfactorily. And yet when it comes to an organizer of the brain's activities, nobody is at home.

o

THE LISTENER

I am not *certain* that anybody is trying to poison me. Obviously, if I was certain about all this, I would do something about it."

At this point my patient, a thirty-seven-year-old businessman (let's call him Dennis) smiles and looks directly at me. But his eyes are far from smiling. Someone could make one wrong move, and this guy, who is a hunter and a marksman, might kill him with one of the guns he keeps in his room at home, I think. A slipup of my own making, and he might decide to terminate our sessions (or perhaps to terminate me).

Two days earlier Dennis came to me convinced that his brain harbored a tumor or "something very definitely wrong." When the tests turned out negative, he finally got around to telling me what was really on his mind: "Something or somebody has to be responsible for all these strange things I am experiencing. The tingling sensation inside my head, the dizziness, the head pain. Somebody is trying to poison me."

Nothing about Dennis's appearance prepares you for anything like that; in fact nothing about him suggests much out of the ordinary. He is tall and well groomed, and wears a suit made more casual by brand-new Hush Puppies. His glasses give him a scholarly appearance, and the frontal balding adds five or ten years to his age. But it's not how he looks that makes him different—it's what he says, how he says it, and what he believes.

Delusions are interesting, elusive, and treacherous to deal with. They pose a real danger for the doctor. Most patients who kill their doctors are motivated by the conviction that the doctor has become part of the problem rather than a means toward its solution. Danger also exists for other people. Dennis is "almost convinced" that his brother, who is three years older and also lives at home, has something to do with the poisoning. "But I'm not really sure. . . . I just think he might be involved." It's that "not really sure" statement that I decide to use in my opening move.

"So you admit there is something about all this that you're unsure about. And you mentioned a moment ago you're not absolutely certain that the poisoning is taking place. How sure are you that you are being poisoned? Give me a percentage between one hundred percent absolute certainty and zero percent certainty that the poisoning is taking place."

"I'd say about ninety-five percent."

"So there's five percent of disbelief here. Five percent of you that says, 'Maybe this isn't happening'?"

"Yeah. . . . I guess so."

Dennis is getting uncomfortable. He's preparing himself for what he thinks is coming: remonstrances, appeals to reason, argumentation.

Somebody once said never to argue with a man with a gun in his hand. He could just as aptly have warned against arguing with somebody with a delusion in his head. That's because if you reason with such a person, particularly if you reason too well, you risk the danger of becoming part of the delusion. Something you say, how you say it, or perhaps something you do that you're not even aware of may suggest to the deluded person that you know more about the delusion than you're telling.

Participation within the delusion—taking the tack "Okay, let's relax. We're all a little crazy now, aren't we?"—is another approach that some doctors try. Personally, I've never been comfortable with it. Certainly I'd have difficulty doing what I once saw on a video monitor: a psychiatrist sitting in his patient's room and discussing with the patient, who was convinced that she was dead, those relatives who had or had not attended her funeral. The most basic problem with such an approach is what it can do to that valuable 5 percent of the patient's mind that hasn't yet gone around the bend. What could be more frightening to that tiny oasis of sanity than learning, from the physician's own words, that the doctor, who is presumably there to help you, is himself unhinged?

Every delusion provides a solution for an uncomfortable internal state. It can be anxiety; more often it's something more subtle: a vague state of uneasiness; something "in the air"; something threatening, yet obscure. The delusion resolves such inner discomforts, but at a price. In a moment that some sufferers have described as one of "great clarity" or profound "insight," the delusional solution emerges like a figure stepping out of a fog bank: "But *of course*. The uneasiness, the fear, and the prickling sensations—someone's trying to poison me!"

Less-dangerous versions of delusion are commonplace. If you enter a room and the conversation ceases and all eyes turn toward you, the thought "Were they talking about me?" immediately springs to mind. This isn't abnormal; everybody is susceptible to such suspicions. The degree of credence given to such thoughts, however, is usually very low. But with individuals like Dennis— reclusive, sensitive, frustrated at not having accomplished more in life, puzzled and perplexed by his inability to understand and anticipate other people's motives—suspicion rapidly escalates into certainty.

Basically the deluded person believes what he does because it somehow *feels right*. As William James pointed out a century ago in an aptly titled essay, "The Sentiment of Rationality," many of our social, political, and moral beliefs rest on a kind of visceral certitude: "I know it in my heart," we say when we are absolutely convinced. We "cross our heart" or raise our right hand as if taking an oath. That certainty originates in the temporal lobes of the

human brain. We know this because epileptics with seizures originating in the temporal lobes often speak of a feeling of "utter
conviction" or "great insight."

In most people this feeling of certainty attaches to generally
accepted ideas and thoughts. But with a delusion an idea that the
person would never have found acceptable under ordinary circumstances can instantly crystallize into certainty. At that moment, the
anxiety, uneasiness, and vague disquietude disappear, to be replaced by an almost blissful state. Naturally, this kind of feeling
isn't relinquished easily—hence the intransigence of the delusional belief. Those who destroy the delusion and thereby threaten
to bring about a restoration of the dreaded doubts, fears, and
anxieties risk becoming the objects of a murderous frenzy.

Dennis is not unusual in wanting to get rid of uncertainties and
anxieties. Nothing could be more natural. The human brain tends
to put the best possible light on things. We have a deeply felt need
to construct explanations about the world and our mental experiences. When it comes to the meaning of events surrounding us, we
abhor uncertainty, ambiguity, being "left hanging."

Remaining reasonably comfortable under conditions of great uncertainty. Rejecting simplistic explanations and premature conclusions. Pressing on in the face of situations that are overdetermined
and ambiguous. These are the qualities of the master tactician, the
warrior, the genius. Unfortunately, they are not qualities that Dennis has in very great supply at the moment.

As Dennis continues to talk, I weigh my options. Forced hospitalization is impossible and most likely unnecessary. Of course,
if he actually kills his brother, then the fact that he did so will
make it easy for some people and their lawyers to conclude that I
could have anticipated and prevented the act. (A little paranoid
delusion of my own, perhaps?) Voluntary hospitalization makes no
sense. Dennis continues to work and doesn't talk to anybody except
me about these things. Besides, there is no drug available that
makes somebody snap out of a delusion and say: "What a crazy
idea *that* was."

No . . . there is only one treatment that has a chance of working with Dennis: Return to the doubt, emphasize the uncertainty, don't judge, don't criticize, don't argue. Most important of all, *keep listening* for every opportunity to enhance and nurture that precious 5 percent of sanity.

POLITICS
AND TEMPERAMENT

Understanding the human brain is such an effective antidote to rigid and inflexible thinking that all those in a position to influence public opinion (all newspaper columnists; talk show hosts; authors, including me; and other self-appointed "social commentators") should be required to study it. They have nothing to lose but their prejudices about human behavior.

For instance, I have never fully understood why many people are offended by the idea that valid deductions about a person's character or personality can be gathered by careful observations of such things as gait, eye color, or bodily proportions. To make such assertions is to risk being accused of being intolerant, racist, and judgmental.

Yet my specialties of neurology and neuropsychiatry are based on the careful observation of such questions as these: Does the patient swing both his arms equally when he walks? (A small stroke or tumor may make its presence known by a reduction in normal arm swing on one side.) Do the facial muscles contract spontaneously and with variation? (Patients with Parkinson's disease display little or no facial movement.) Is the person overly concrete in his thinking? ("What brought you to the hospital today?" is the first question a doctor asks to get the patient to talk about his problems. "I came on the bus," answer schizophrenics and sufferers from certain forms of brain damage.)

My concern here can be summed up concisely: biological observations are pertinent to patients suffering from neurologic and psychiatric illnesses. Why, then, wouldn't a similar approach be useful in trying to understand human behavior in general? Jerome Kagan, a psychologist at Harvard University, provides an answer to this question: social and political preconceptions work to separate environmental factors from biological ones.

> *A good number of American psychologists would like to believe that, regardless of children's genotypes, it should be possible to discover environmental manipulations that will produce equally competent children and adults. The possibility that some genotypes are more and some less malleable to a given class of experience implies an unfair constraint on benevolent intervention, even though no one believes it's possible to make a wolf as relaxed as a beagle.*

Kagan's reference to a beagle will strike a note in anyone who has kept dogs. The nervous fretfulness of my Pekingese couldn't be more different from the stable, unflappable demeanor of my neighbor's bulldog. Nor is the gentleness of the collie I knew as a child likely to be found in a pit bull purchased and trained for aggression to satisfy its owner's paranoid fantasies. The research done by the Russian experimental physiologist Ivan Pavlov verifies our intuition that dogs possess distinct personalities.

In one Pavlov-inspired experiment a circle was used as a conditioning stimulus to inform a dog that it would be fed; the presence of an ellipse indicated no food would be forthcoming. Barely perceptible alterations made the ellipse more and more like a circle. Finally, when the ellipse was nearly indistinguishable from a circle, the dog indicated its understanding of the change by lining up for its food.

After a few weeks of constantly having to make these subtle distinctions, the dogs became, in Pavlov's word, "neurotic": excitable, agitated, no longer able to distinguish between obvious circles and ellipses. He called the animals' reaction an experimental neurosis and blamed it on a disturbance in the balance between excitatory and inhibitory processes in the nervous system. Pavlov also noticed something that had escaped other researchers: dogs with different personalities responded in different ways to the same experiment. In other words, the same treatment (animal rights groups might prefer the word *mistreatment*) when applied to different dogs produced different neuroses.

Applications of Pavlov's findings of temperamental differences among dogs have never really been very enthusiastically received in the United States. Many of us are convinced that biology should mirror our social and political beliefs rather than the other way around. For instance, several years ago neuroscientists began to speak about differences in the brains of men and women. This immediately caused such an uproar (one researcher, Edward Wilson, had a pitcher of water poured over his head during a lecture in Boston) that neuroscientists largely gave up on the subject. To speak of brain sex differences—worse yet, to demonstrate them— was to have one's contribution considered another brick in the wall of sexism that has made women's lives so difficult for so long. At least that is the fear expressed by many people. It's also a concern one hears frequently from talk show hosts, editorial writers, and others who influence popular opinion. After all, ours is an egalitarian country where not only should every dog have its day, but every dog should be equal to every other dog. That is, although you might accept that your Labrador may be a better companion on a duck hunting expedition than your prissy poodle, you would certainly bristle at the suggestion that those differences might be based on any weakness in the poodle's nervous system. At least that's how you would respond if your thinking is in sync with the traditional overemphasis on the environment as the determining influence on behavior.

Most of us can't accept that dogs exhibit temperamental differences based on the organization of their brains. So it's no mystery why differences of temperament within our own species are resisted with the self-righteous vigor of a Bible Belt preacher presented with an issue of *Hustler*. We, as a society, have decided that information about temperament, however interesting it sounds, is potentially too divisive and controversial to be tolerated.

All of which makes Kagan and his associates' findings on temperament, especially what they refer to as "inhibited children," even more interesting and provocative. They have identified a small group of fearful, timid infants (perhaps one in ten or fifteen) who grow into anxious adolescents and later shy, cautious adults given to anxiety and even periodic attacks of panic. These inhibited children are distinguishable by their birth order, physical appearance, behavior, and physiology. In general, they are born later, are blue-eyed, and display a lowered threshold for arousal within the portions of the brain important in processing fear and anxiety (the limbic hypothalamic areas).

Kagan based his criteria for limbic arousal largely on measurements of activity within the sympathetic nervous system, originating from the limbic hypothalamic areas. Included were changes in heart rate, pupillary dilatation, and norepinephrine blood levels in response to psychological stress and challenge. Kagan also included measurements of muscle tension and the levels of neurotransmitters and endocrine secretions within blood, saliva, and urine. The pooled research revealed a substantial positive relationship between the research findings and the behavioral trait of inhibition.

"We suggest, albeit speculatively, that most of the children we call inhibited belong to a qualitatively distinct category of infants who were born with a lower threshold for limbic hypothalamic arousal to unexpected changes in the environment or novel events that cannot be assimilated easily," Kagan concluded.

About now you are probably wondering, "So what? Everybody knows that kids don't respond the same way to the same experiences. Is there anything so revolutionary about the idea that some of this might be based on brain differences"?

Indeed there is. Psychologists and psychiatrists have been arguing for decades over the existence of innate behavior traits—in other words, temperament. Freud spoke of libidinal energy, but never accepted the claims of his disciple Carl Jung that people possess nervous systems that vary from weak to strong. Jung claimed, for instance, that more intense primary forces exist within the introvert. That's why introverts appear more tense, often over-react, and take longer periods to recover from upsetting experiences. Conversely, the extrovert's brain possesses a "higher restitutive capacity" than the introvert's.

On a more practical level Jung believed, in contrast to Freud, that temperamental factors contribute to such things as social anxiety, avoidance reactions, panic attacks, and agoraphobia. (Freud classified those conditions as results of hysteria, a term with very little current cachet.)

Over the decades Jung has turned out to be something of a prophet. His speculations about introverts' requiring a longer time to recover from stress agrees almost exactly with Kagan's findings that inhibited children display a greater arousal of the sympathetic and hypothalamic pituitary adrenal axis following certain stresses. Such children also require a longer recovery time than uninhibited children.

These new and exciting findings are not confined to inhibited behavior, introversion, or qualitative responses to stress. The brain, it appears, is important in other behavioral areas as well. Obsessions and compulsions are now believed to be the result of disturbances in the basal ganglia, several structures lying beneath the cerebral hemispheres. And PET scans show distinctive patterns in some cases of schizophrenia and manic depression. Hyperactivity and dyslexia, too, can be diagnosed on the basis of brain maps—computer-assisted EEGs—that show atypical brain areas involved in reading or writing. It's likely that soon these brain maps may be as unique as fingerprints. But what's to be done now about all of the presumably well-meaning but misguided people who can't seem to keep their biology separated from their politics?

"There has always been, as there is now, a tension in Western views toward the origin of psychological differences and desire, supported by commitment to egalitarianism, to minimize biology and maximize experience," as Kagan puts it. How to best present neurological insights about human nature without arousing fierce opposition creates a dilemma, one that isn't going to be easy to resolve. As a first step, it would help if all statements about biological contributions to behavior were not interpreted as disguised fascism. The resulting insights into ourselves might be liberating rather than limiting.

This is particularly important for people in the media. Reporters and commentators should periodically remind themselves that not every scientist who claims that her research indicates a biological origin for certain behaviors or for intelligence or for emotional development should be labeled a racist. It might be more useful to look at the evidence, to review the data and the arguments analytically. It's never wise to allow our political instincts to dictate our views of new discoveries about the brain and behavior. As an unexpected benefit to that approach toward new knowledge, we may learn a lot of liberating rather than limiting things about ourselves.

As for myself, I find brain-based insights about temperament rather comforting. For one thing, I no longer have to despair that as much as I might wish otherwise, I, along with some of my best friends, fit into that inhibited category.

But, after all, things could be worse: I could have been born *uninhibited* and, by this time, have inflicted untold mischief upon the world.

An *uninhibited* neuropsychiatrist on the loose and in practice. Now *there's* a devil of an idea to conjure with. . . .

o

DREAM PUZZLES

Several years ago, sleep and dream researcher William Dement gave the following problem to five hundred Stanford University undergraduates: The letters O, T, T, F, F . . . form the beginning of an infinite sequence. Find a simple rule for determining any or all successive letters. According to your rule, what would be the next two letters of the sequence?

The students were then asked to write down any dreams they had the next night. The correct solution to the problem appeared in seven dreams, but none of the seven students had reached the correct answer to the problem prior to the dream.

One of the students who solved the problem in a dream gave this account: "I was standing in an art gallery, looking at the paintings on the wall. As I walked down the hall, I began to count the paintings: one, two, three, four, five. As I came to the sixth and seventh, the paintings had been ripped from their frames. I stared at the empty frames with a peculiar feeling that some mystery was about to be solved. Suddenly I realized that the sixth and seventh spaces were the solution to the problem!"

The solution to the problem is that O, T, T, F, F are the first letters of *One, Two, Three, Four, Five*. Obviously the next letters are S and S, standing for *Six* and *Seven*, and so on. But the dream raises questions far more important and intriguing than just the solution to the puzzle: At what point did the solution occur to the dreamer? Did it happen at the start, when the dreamer actually began counting the paintings, thus intuitively realizing that *counting* would lead to the solution? Or was it when the dreamer encountered two empty frames, which represents the problem of five known letters and two unknown ones?

At a deeper level of analysis lies the question "Who came up with the answer?" The response "The dreamer did, of course," begs an important question: The student could not arrive at an answer by conscious, wakeful reflection, but could do so in a dream, albeit in a disguised form. Does this mean that the student actually knew the answer to the problem but couldn't come up with that answer for some reason? In short, did he actually know that he knew it? Or was the solution actually worked out within the dream? If you prefer this last explanation, then what does it say about the organization of the human brain that problem solving can be more effective in a state of profound unconsciousness than in full, concentrated alertness?

John Cohen, emeritus professor of psychology at the University of Manchester, encourages us to think of the mind as a self-communicating system: "Introspection is the best known example of self communicating, but this takes place at the surface, as it were," writes Cohen. "There are species of what we might describe as 'subterranean' self-communication in which we tell things to ourselves, or inquire from ourselves. That indescribably complex entity that we call the 'self' has 1,000 ways of 'reflection,' through dreams and reverie, and many physiological indices of revelation, betrayal or intimation, such as blushing, trembling, growing pale or panicky, or collapsing. Indeed, the whole gambit of emotion is a means of self-communion."

As an example of this self-communion, consider this dream told to me by a married patient who was having an affair with a recently divorced woman. Over the past several weeks my patient had worried about acts of carelessness by his lover that could have led to his wife's discovery of the liaison:

"My girlfriend and I were lying on a beach together. Suddenly I heard the sound of a car headed toward us. I looked up from the blanket and spotted a familiar-looking sports car headed along the beach at a rapid speed. As the car neared, I recognized it as my girlfriend's sports car. I also recognized, to my terror, that the car was headed directly toward us and to avoid injury or death we would have to move quickly. Just at the moment I was turning to warn my girlfriend, I took one final look at the approaching car. To my terror, I recognized that my girlfriend was at the wheel at the same time she was lying on the blanket beside me."

The dreamer awoke startled and filled with anxiety. At that moment he understood that the destructive unconscious purpose behind his girlfriend's recent carelessness was to bring about discovery of the liaison and break up the dreamer's marriage. The danger implicit in such an enterprise was conveyed by the image of the girlfriend: she was both an active agent in bringing about the eventual confrontation (she was the driver of the car) and a potential victim with the dreamer of the consequences of the discovery of their affair (she was at the same time lying asleep on the beach next to her lover).

The solution to my patient's dilemma occurred, as with the dream of Dement's student, in an image one step removed from the verbal explanation. In both instances a vivid visual scenario held the key to the solution of a baffling problem. The conscious part of the mind wrestled with the problem but could not come up with the solution until another part, completely cut off from conscious deliberation, produced a disguised solution in the form of an image.

More precisely, the mind seems to operate here as an assembly of associated subunits, each unit informing the other. Out of that interplay of subunits emerges a unification that isn't the product of any one of them. The solutions to the problems arise not as the result of an exercise in reasoning, but "out of the blue," almost as if the solutions had been provided by someone else. But there does not seem to be an overall writer, producer, or director who consciously controls the plot. Such a distributed information system can now be directly visualized, thanks to PET scans.

In one of the experiments of neurophysiologist Per Roland, the subject is instructed to detect a very weak touch at the tip of the index finger. However, no touch or other stimulus is actually delivered. Nonetheless, expectation and the pure focusing of attention on an index fingertip increases cerebral blood flow in the sensory hand area, the anterior and midpoint of the superior frontal cortex, the midfrontal cortex, and the sensory association areas. Awareness and conscious attention is thus widely distributed throughout the brain. Further, since no sensory information is delivered—no touch—the resulting pattern, corresponding to a pure thought, is the result of the brain's own widespread organizational activity. The focused attention that is subjectively experienced as a unity is actually the result of the synchrony of many brain areas.

But who or what is doing the organizing? The traditional response, "I make the decision, which my brain carries out for me," simply won't do in light of organizational activities taking place prior to conscious awareness.

In "Your Brain Has a Mind of Its Own" I discussed Benjamin Libet's research that led to the discovery of an electrical change within the brain that occurs up to half a second before the subject mentally decides to make a movement: the brain begins to work *before* a subject's conscious intention to act.

Libet's and Roland's work suggests changing the traditional response from "I decide, and my brain executes my decision" to "I am my brain; my brain and I are one." It is futile to think of oneself as anything other than or in any way distinct from one's brain.

The work of the neurologist Richard Jung offers a fascinating example of this concept.

First Jung attaches electrodes to a volunteer's head and to muscles at various parts of the body. That way Jung can study the sequence of events that occur as the subject carries out a spontaneous voluntary movement. At this point the volunteer is instructed to punch out at a target at a moment of his own choosing. The sequence involves ten recordable events, only two of which are consciously directed. The other eight consisted of unconscious coordinations: preparatory balancing movements, a preparatory movement of the eyes, bodily rotation, postural movements in the muscles of the trunk and legs, and so on.

In Jung's experiment, to ask "Who is doing the organizing?" implies a persona, a homunculus, a self. Yet Libet's, Roland's, and Jung's findings suggest something far less unified, something along the lines of a committee of selves, or what split brain researcher Michael Gazzaniga calls a "confederacy of mental systems."

Gazzaniga speaks of our mental lives as amounting to a "reconstruction of the independent activities of the many brain systems we all possess."

In evaluating the insights provided by research on the human brain, how does one answer the question "Who am I?" One thing is certain: there is no simple, logically compelling answer. The poet W. H. Auden intuitively grasped this dilemma:

"Who am I? Several answers are possible, but there can no more be one definitive answer than there can be one definitive history of the Thirty Years' War."

What better way to experience this confederacy of selves, therefore, than by solving problems while dreaming? Here's one final one, also from Dement: Consider the letters *H, I, J, K, L, M, N, O.* This sequence should suggest one word. What is that word? If you can't figure it out while awake and concentrating, you might wish to solve it by remembering your dreams.

One dreamer reported, "I had several dreams, all of which had water in them somewhere. In one dream I was hunting sharks. In another I was confronted by a barracuda while skin diving. In another dream it was raining heavily. In another I was sailing into the wind."

Given that report, can you come up with the one-word solution? (No points for sequence or alphabet. Dement refused to accept either as correct.) The dreamer knew the answer; indeed, he represented it repeatedly in the dream images.

The answer? Water, of course: the sequence of letters proceeds from H to O, i.e., H_2O. One area of the dreamer's brain knew the answer but wasn't telling that part of the brain involved in introspection and self-report. It's difficult to think that this arrangement expresses self-unity. Closer to the facts is psychologist John Cohen's definition: "The self is a hierarchical structure of sub-selves, an organization of elements in a more or less constant state of internal tussle."

Perhaps if Shakespeare had known what we now know about our deductive powers in a dream state, he would have written: "To sleep, perhaps to dream . . . and thereby solve."

o

BYTES
ON THE BRAIN

I s the human brain losing ground to computers? Many computer scientists and artificial intelligence experts believe so.
But before uncritically accepting this gloomy prospect, consider these differences.

Each living brain cell, or neuron, is altered by its experiences
and its environment. And since each cell influences the action of
another, it becomes that much easier for the same response to
occur a second time. This is the basis for habit. But in contrast to
computers, brains can alter their habitual responses, sometimes
with difficulty—e.g., when we learn to refrain from that second
piece of pie. At the nerve cell level this involves a lessening of the
tendency for neurons to set up reverberating networks that represent the desire for that second piece of pie.

Computer chips, in contrast, aren't alive, don't spontaneously
reorganize themselves, don't undertake their own modifications in
their functioning.

Computers, in general, are designed to deal with information
presented one bit at a time (serially), while brains operate via the
use of subsystems that function in tandem (parallel processing).

As an example of parallel processing, consider that at the same
time you can read this essay, drink your coffee without spilling it,
listen for the sound of the toaster, and monitor the weather report
on the radio that drones on in the background. Parallel inputs, in

short, present little difficulty for brains; but only the most recent, expensive, and sophisticated computers are capable of significant parallel processing.

Neurons, contrasted with computers, don't operate according to a binary code (off/on). Whether one brain cell fires depends upon the influence of perhaps thousands of other cells that make contact with it. Subtract several hundred inhibitory influences from the neuron, and it may fire. The same result can be produced by adding several hundred excitatory influences. The neuron, in short, is always in a dynamic state that alters within thousandth-of-a-second intervals.

What one nerve cell "tells" the next depends upon the "conversation" going on between hundreds, and in some cases thousands, of cells separated by varying distances. Put another way, nerve cell communication depends upon the establishment of networks, or cell assemblies.

"Any two cells or systems of cells which are repeatedly active at the same time will tend to become 'associated' so that activity in one facilitates activity in the other," wrote neurophysiologist Donald Hebb in 1949 in perhaps this century's most important book on the brain, *The Organization of Behavior.*

Nothing like this exists within computers, which is one of the reasons that a nine-month-old infant can recognize her mother, while a computer capable of specific facial recognition is only the stuff of science fiction.

As another way of putting it, the brain's functional capacities are distributed. This means that if one part breaks down, another part can be recruited to take its place. Any failure of performance resulting from this arrangement is distinctly human. "You know, he was the guy that ran a peanut farm before he was president," we may say when we're on the right track but can't quite come up with the name of Jimmy Carter. "Graceful degradation" is the whimsical term for this loss of clarity and precision. We exhibit it (or, rather, our brains do), but computers don't. They can't. A computer either comes up with the specific information requested or doesn't. It is not good at recognizing alternative ways of signifying the same thing. But the brain is good at it, a facility made possible by the cell assemblies just mentioned.

If a sufficient number of cell assemblies are coupled together, generalizations become possible that are beyond even the most sophisticated computer. For instance, we recognize a Chippendale chair, a sofa, an empty orange crate, and a tree stump as things to sit on. This recognition is based on many cell assemblies involving thousands, perhaps even millions, of neurons' overlapping to form a meta-assembly that is responsible for the abstract concept.

The greater diversity of the brain, contrasted with a computer, also depends, to a large extent, on the fact that the brain is a "wet organ"; that is, it employs chemicals known as neurotransmitters (also sometimes called regulatory hormones) in order to transmit its signals. In contrast, the computer is as dry as dust. It's the difference between a hormonally driven gland (the brain) and an electrically driven device (the computer).

The brain's regulatory hormones (more than thirty are known at the moment) are thought to function like the letters of the alphabet. Every English sentence written is composed using only these twenty-six letters. The number of possible combinations of letters approaches infinity, but only some combinations will be meaningful; others are only strings of letters that add up to nonsense.

The challenge for neuroscientists is to discover which combinations of neurotransmitters and regulatory hormones are functionally active. In an allied challenge, scientists must discover what they do. Some facilitate communication and neuronal firing. Others are inhibitory. Many of the hormones are locally active, while others influence nerve cells great distances away.

What is really astonishing about neurons, and what sets them firmly apart from computer components, is that they can change their chemical identity. A neuron may cease to employ its usual neurotransmitter in favor of another. Or neurotransmitters and hormones that regulate actions at the synapse may start working in concert. In this way one neurotransmitter can be responsible for fast chemical signaling between neurons, while the second transmitter will mediate slower, more diffuse changes in functioning.

As another point of difference from computers, neurotransmitters and regulatory hormones are not restricted to the brain. They can be found in such places as the intestines, the lungs, and the sexual organs. This ubiquity has stimulated a startling question that is currently haunting neuroscientists around the world: Is it possible that our definition of the brain is too narrow? That the regulatory processes we now localize within our heads are much more widely distributed?

As a result of their research, many neuroscientists now believe that the brain is not like a computer or a machine, at least not like any machine that anyone has ever encountered. It has no definable boundaries (neuroregulatory hormones are dispersed throughout the body). Its parts can break down through disuse or mishap, and yet its functioning may not be perceptively altered. For example, we're losing neurons throughout our lifetime (about fifty thousand cells per day, about ten thousand synapses per second), yet our mental capacities improve, or at least hold steady, until late in our lives.

In addition, the brain's status as a wet organ endows it with the capacity to communicate by releasing chemicals into the environment that act at sites other than the synapse.

But if the brain is not like a computer, then what is it like? What kind of model can we form in regard to its functioning? I believe there's only one answer to that question, and perhaps it will disturb you: *there is no model of the brain, nor will there ever be.* That's because the brain, as the constructor of all models, transcends all models. The brain's uniqueness stems from the fact that nowhere in the known universe is there anything even remotely resembling it. So rest easy. Although computers and neuronal networks may challenge us, amuse us, even extend our intellectual horizons, they will never, ever replace us.

PRESCRIPTIONS
FOR INSIGHT

I often wonder what hope there can be for troubled people who can't obtain professional help. It seems unfair that individually and collectively we've become increasingly dependent on psychiatrists, psychologists, and social workers—professions that a century ago didn't exist, at least in their present forms. What did our ancestors do with their angst?

Although conventional wisdom has it that less-complicated times bred less-complicated emotional disturbances, I find this hard to believe. Love and jealousy and low self-esteem and sadness didn't originate with the telephone or the radio: they are aspects of the universal human condition, and *that* has lasted quite a long time on this planet.

One has only to read the Greek tragedies, Shakespeare, or Dickens to see that people have been trying for centuries to cope with uncomfortable feelings, distressing thoughts, and uncontrollable impulses. Today, of course, the person afflicted with these disturbances is encouraged to visit a psychiatrist or a psychoanalyst. Isn't it interesting in that regard that Sigmund Freud, the most famous analyst of all, was himself never analyzed? Interesting, too, that some of the most mixed-up people around—I am talking here not of definable mental illness, but of people who seem normal enough to all outward appearances yet can't seem to get their lives together—are regular consumers of psychiatric help. Instead of helping them, however, psychiatric treatment has only deepened their narcissism. They can't wait to tell you, again and again and again, how therapy is helping them to get deeply in touch with their own feelings. Translation: They have become so totally self-absorbed that they have lost all sensitivity to the feelings of others. For these people the need for perpetual therapy has become a part of the problem, instead of one step toward a solution. Perhaps Freud was thinking of them when he wrote of analysis terminable and interminable. If so, the people I am speaking about here have opted for the latter.

Of course, there are avenues for self-exploration other than psychiatry or psychoanalysis. The number of self-help books increases every year. But life isn't lived between the covers of a book. And I've yet to meet anyone who has maintained for more than a few weeks his initial claim that a certain self-help book has "changed my life."

For those who aren't fond of reading, communal exercises in self-help are available. EST and Lifespring and other touchy-feely therapies glorify the blessings one can expect from declarations of self-worth and becoming "totally honest" about one's feelings. They also encourage a lot of hugging and "affirming" of other people making the same journey toward self-discovery and fulfillment. But these communal group grope approaches also seem to work only for a little while. Perhaps it has something to do with the fact that it's hard to maintain continuity by spilling out your most intimate thoughts to people you will never see again after the weekend.

And then there's the most perilous avenue of all: self-revelation to friends. For reasons that I've never understood, people who are extremely circumspect in other aspects of their lives oftentimes readily reveal intimate and potentially dangerous disclosures about their private lives (usually affairs) to friends who they know from experience can't be trusted to keep a secret. "Flooders" is the marvelously apt term used by psychologists to refer to these people, perhaps driven by guilt, for whom problems and complexes gush out from every pore, drowning the listener and usually ending the friendship.

"When a good friend starts telling me something too personal or that smacks too much of a therapy situation, I try as tactfully as I can to convey the message 'Please don't.' That's because for me the friendship has to end when I no longer can just listen, but find myself judging or criticizing or even blaming that person for her problems." That's how one woman I know handles the flooder. Granted, she may sound more superficial than compassionate; but at least she knows her limitations as an amateur psychotherapist. Most important, she is acutely tuned in to her low level of tolerance for hearing about other people's problems.

What, then, is one to do about personal angst in place of psychiatric treatment, self-help books, group experiences, and overwhelming our friends with self-revelations? A psychiatrist friend who to all outward appearances at least seems well adapted made the following suggestions: If the goal is learning more about yourself, then who knows more about you than yourself? Therefore, keep a journal. Write down over a ten-minute period every day everything that occurs to you in that short period of time. The goal is to keep the pen moving as fast as you can. Don't stop or hesitate, no matter what appears on the paper. Fantasies, daydreams, statements of discouragement about what you're doing at that moment, grocery lists—it doesn't matter. Just keep writing. After the ten-minute exercise, take another ten minutes, and this time write in a more recollective mode. Monitor consciously, clearly, and even a bit critically what you're going to write at the moment you write it. When finished, put the journal away until the next day. Repeat this exercise for several weeks without reading any of the previous entries. You will benefit from seeing your thoughts and feelings written out in tangible form. This reality is an important step toward achieving the primary goal of any insight therapy: a sense of objectivity about yourself.

Moreover, the journal entries provide the opportunity to notice if ideas, fantasies, and moods recur, and if they create any kind of pattern. Be forewarned that patterns won't be noticed except over the long haul and only if, as suggested, you can refrain from the understandable but ultimately stifling tendency to read previous entries. If you can do this, you may be surprised to learn that your moods and impulses often follow repetitive patterns. That knowledge alone will probably place you in the top 1 percent of psychologically sophisticated people. Most of us remain blissfully and tragically unaware that the same patterns of difficulty recur again and again. Because of this, they rarely prove any more manageable the nth time around.

As a second method of self-analysis, buy a watch with an alarm on it. Have a friend set the alarm for random moments during the day. Obviously, since you didn't set the alarm, you will have no idea when the alarm will go off. When it does, immediately write down what you are thinking and how you feel at *that instant*. This method, known as thought tracking, gets around most of the customary defensive maneuvers. You'll get a direct view of your mental contents and mood at a specific moment not of your choosing. That is a lot more spontaneous and existentially valid than any recollection drawn from your memory hours or days later when you're talking to a psychiatrist.

Dreams, despite a lot of nonsense written about them, also provide valuable self-insights. But for reasons known only to Mother Nature, dreams aren't usually retained by our brain in retrievable form so that we can recall them in the morning. Indeed, self-reports from patients and others seem to suggest some people don't dream at all. But J. Allen Hobson assures me that almost all of us do dream and that in most instances our dreaming can be increased if we simply decide to start dreaming more. The whole process takes about three weeks and is easy to execute. Simply be determined—"Tonight I am going to dream, and I'll remember my dream"—and the remembering becomes fairly automatic after that.

Once the dreams start, get a tape recorder and keep it by your bedside. When you awaken in the morning, dictate everything that you can remember about what you dreamed during the night. This record, like the journal, should be consulted only at infrequent intervals.

Daydreams are even more helpful in achieving insight, but are limited by the difficulties most of us have in capturing them. Since daydreams occur in a state closely akin to reverie, our critical faculties are usually at a low ebb. Indeed, to simultaneously be aware of a daydream and at the same time critique it requires a split in consciousness that not all of us can achieve.

Random, seemingly "crazy" associations that spring to mind at odd moments during the day can also provide clues to inner themes and scenarios that we may be consciously unaware of. For instance, on one occasion a vivid image came to me of my wife and President Bush holding hands in the Rose Garden. By tossing the image about in the air with some playfulness, I discovered the theme: both my wife and President Bush are left-handed, and both had recently done something I considered clumsy, or gauche. Further, in an earlier discussion on a political subject, my wife had, to my surprise, defended the president—thus allying herself with him, a union signified by the image of their hand-holding.

Thoughts are always associated with subtle and not-so-subtle emotional feelings. That's because within the brain the areas mediating thoughts and feelings are intricately interconnected. In fact, it's almost impossible to have a thought without at the same time having some feeling about it. On some occasions, the feelings are as evanescent and subtle as sunlight playing on gently moving water. But with some practice it's possible to be swift enough to tune in to these feelings. Often they take the form of bodily sensations: a vague sense of "heaviness" somewhere in the chest or legs or head, migraine headaches, a problem with getting one's breath, and so on. These positive and emotional reactions can tell us a lot about ourselves. With practice comes a talent for registering and recognizing our own moods and responses without the usual self-judging and self-criticism. This agrees with what Zen masters have suggested over the centuries: that the mind is a blue sky, and our thoughts and emotions are like clouds that appear against that sky and then disappear. *Mindfulness* consists in observing those clouds—our thoughts and emotions—while remaining confident that no matter what their form or content, our thoughts and emotions, like the clouds, will soon disappear, leaving once again only the blueness of the sky.

Last, a word of caution: None of the methods I've described is guaranteed to enable one to accomplish that most difficult of all feats of self-analysis, control of one's own mind. Nevertheless, I am convinced that they *can* help. Doesn't the only real mind control worth achieving come from observing our own mental reactions and learning as much as possible about them?

o

IS RUGGED INDIVIDUALISM EXTINCT?

Recent studies indicate that manic depression and Alzheimer's disease may be associated with genetic abnormalities at specific sites along the human chromosome. The good news is that treatments using genetic engineering may soon be available to help prevent these diseases. The bad news is that most of us aren't comfortable with genetic explanations for our own or anyone else's behavior. We are proud of our freedom, individuality, and powers of self-determination; therefore, the notion that complex behaviors such as manic depression and Alzheimer's are genetically preordained isn't terribly popular. Our reluctance stems from the implicit belief that our behavior must involve something nonphysical, some aspect of the human spirit.

We know that the brain is the organ responsible for the operation of the mind, but we want to believe that this organ is somehow different from, say, the kidney, the liver, or the lungs. We do this despite suggestions to the contrary that can be traced back at least as far as the Greeks.

"Not only our pleasure, our joy, and our laughter, but also our sorrow, pain, grief, and tears arise from the brain and the brain alone," wrote Hippocrates, the legendary father of medicine. "With it we think and understand, see and hear, and we distinguish between the ugly and the beautiful, between what is pleasant and what is unpleasant, and between good and evil."

If behavior is based on our own genes, then our freedom, so the reasoning goes, may be largely illusory. We will be at the mercy of circumstances and whim; a Calvinistic determinism will preordain our fate.

We tend to resist scientific findings that emphasize the importance of inheritance or genetic traits over self-determination. Our freewheeling individualism is vaguely affronted by the prospect that Uncle Jim's alcoholism might bear some relation to the depression that at certain moments tugs at our innards. Granted that our depression may manifest itself in mood swings or psychic inertia rather than in an addiction to drink. But the mechanism is the same in us as it was in Uncle Jim—the blues.

A lifetime spent in a democratic society in which everyone is equal before the law makes it only too easy to conclude that everyone is also equal biologically, that inheritance isn't very important when it comes to diseases of the body and mind. Nothing could be further from the truth. Modern genetics, especially the work on Alzheimer's and manic depression mentioned earlier, suggests that biologically we remain part of a larger grouping for as long as we live; when it comes to the illnesses that plague us, nobody stands alone.

This insight requires a reordering of priorities in a society such as ours where, for instance, very few people are able to provide their physicians with a family history. I first noticed this several years ago with regard to migraine headaches. Almost without exception, migraines run in families. Other, more serious causes of headache can often be eliminated from consideration in patients with a strong history of migraines. But few patients these days keep sufficiently in touch with their families to be able to state with any assurance whether or not other family members suffer from migraine headaches. Family members have become somewhat of an embarrassment—people we are related to, but with whom we feel little sense of kinship, mostly good for small talk at weddings and funerals.

But now, thanks to the insights provided by genetics, all this dedication to rugged individualism and isolation may have to change. Biology always places constraints on our freedom. Our need for complete control and absolute autonomy is only a narcissistic self-gratification—the demands of a spoiled child railing against the restraints that prevent him from doing only as he pleases. Moreover, manic depression and Alzheimer's are just the beginning. Many other behaviors are presently under analysis based on studies of adopted children, identical twins, and biochemical profiles. Those of us drawn to simplistic approaches to complex issues will undoubtedly be tempted to try to force these new insights into outmoded arguments: free will versus determinism, fate versus responsibility, heredity versus the environment, and so on. But the new findings render all these once sacred dichotomies irrelevant. Neuroscientific evidence suggests the brain is both partially hard-wired (the newborn infant's impulse to turn toward the source of a sound, especially the mother's voice, is universal) and partially plastic (e.g., our lifelong capability of learning any one of many possible languages, depending on which languages we are exposed to).

The findings concerning manic depression are probably typical of what we can expect to discover about other behavioral disorders. Despite the importance of genetics, environment still plays a role in hereditary illness. As a result of their genetic constitution, some individuals may be strongly predisposed toward mood swings. But even the most biologically predisposed of these individuals may not develop the illness if the environment proves not too stressful. At the other extreme are those with less genetic loading who may sink into despair, depression, and suicide in response to overwhelming rejections, disappointments, or losses. Depression, therefore, should be considered something like the blur we've come to associate with the path of an electron rather than something immutable, like the table upon which I am writing this essay. Our response to manic depression and other behavioral idiosyncrasies will have to adapt to reflect this conceptual change. For the moment, our responses are overly simplistic. For instance, if a child cannot sit still in a classroom, then she may be medicated into submission instead of placed in a less physically inhibiting classroom environment. If an individual is suffering from psychosomatic illness resulting from stress, then many feel that the stress should be managed by tranquilizers instead of by encouraging the worker to ask himself the simple question, "Is this job really worth all this?"

Equally simplistic are contentions such as "There's no crime, only disease," and "No personal responsibility, only an understandable response to a deprived social environment." Because the world is more complicated than most of us can cope with, we seek comfort from clichés and scapegoats. We don't want to hear that there is no single or monolithic solution to some of our most pressing problems: drugs, crime, mental illness, anomie. We can't accept the fact that the old platitudes just don't work anymore. Is mental illness a matter of mind or brain? It's both. Is nature or nurture more important in understanding personality and character? Both are important; neither makes sense without reference to the other. Never has there existed a gene without an environment.

The seemingly important questions of one era aren't so much resolved as they are rendered irrelevant by new information and new findings. No generation has all the answers. That's the uneasy conclusion each of us is going to have to learn to become comfortable with if we are serious about creating a society more humane for the individual and more civilized for the world at large. Rugged individualism still has its place, but total freedom is no longer realistic, workable, or desirable. And I say good riddance—we'll all be better off for it.

o

MIND FLIGHT

The sign on the office door says Mind World. Once inside, visitors plunk down twenty-five dollars, put on goggles and headphones, and then lie back in large reclining chairs to listen to new age music while their eyes are bombarded with colored lights. The machine is called the whole brain wave synchro-energizer. It is said to provide the opportunity for flight into the inner self.

On one occasion I tried such a mind flight. As I lay with my eyes closed, the blinking lights from the goggles produced pulsing colors: red, white, yellow, but mostly purple. At times the colors ran together into tweedlike patterns that revolved kaleidoscopically. As the music began to pulse, the light flashed in synchrony. Interspersed with all of this were sounds of rippling water or bird calls. After a few minutes of this kind of thing, you begin to feel like you're living completely within your skull. It's the ultimate Cartesian dream: *you*, starkly present and aware; and *everything else*, which, while you're on the mind machine, seems much less interesting.

After only a few minutes on the machine I experienced a pleasant floating feeling: the "flight to inner space," as the Mind World people refer to it.

Promised benefits from "frequent flyer" ventures inward include a more relaxed frame of mind, enhanced energy, and improved

130

memory. And also a change in "the quality of one's brain waves, putting them into a more synchronous pattern," as one proponent of the machine puts it. But before you get to that point, you must deal with the light-sound show produced by the synergizer. In my case, as the music picked up in tempo—correlated with whirling, flashing lights and high-flying beeps and heartbeats (definitely not my own)—I started to get uneasy, then uncomfortable. Finally I was afflicted with the "can't get my breath sensation" that happens on a crowded elevator when somebody says, "Hey . . . the door doesn't seem to want to open."

My problem, to be quite candid, is a fear of the contents of my own mind. After some forty years of repression and conformity, I am certain that all kinds of chained and muzzled demons lurk in the murky outer banks of my brainscape. Over the years the rational parts of my brain have managed to establish an uneasy truce with these creepy-crawly denizens who periodically announce their hidden presence through such means as particularly disturbing nightmares. What's true for me holds true, I expect, for others as well. For many of us, uneasy symbiotic alliances—secret sharers—exist within the mind. Their existence may not even be suspected by our consciousness.

Deep below our cerebral hemispheres brain circuits exist that haven't changed much in thousands of years. Destroy all, or portions, of the cerebral cortex and its connection with that deeper-lying and ancient limbic system in an animal such as, say, a hamster, and eerie things begin to happen. Paul MacLean, the world's foremost living researcher on the limbic system, finds that destruction of an area, the cingulate gyrus, which connects the limbic system to the cerebral cortex, produces severe defects in maternal behavior (only 12 percent of pups in a litter survive). "It was as though the animals with the additional loss of cingulate cortex had regressed in the direction of reptiles," MacLean writes.

If you've ever been present during somebody's bad trip on LSD, you've observed firsthand the terror of a person suddenly finding himself one-on-one with a personal demon of his own. Crack and

PCP can do the same thing; they chemically disconnect the limbic system from the controlling cerebral hemispheres. What happens next? Ask any member of the Los Angeles Police Department. You'll learn that it's not unusual for the LAPD to send out a dozen officers to subdue an average-size person on PCP. Such overwhelming force is necessary because this horrific chemical has unleashed a monster from the depths of the brainscape; and as in one of those scenes of mayhem from *King Kong*, there's no reasoning with such a brutally powerful force.

When the restraining influence of our cerebral hemispheres is diminished by drugs or alcohol, the result is rarely an increase in tenderness, thoughtfulness, or connectedness to others. Is this because we're basically violent, murderous creatures whose propensities must continually be controlled and suppressed by our higher brain centers? Or was Rousseau correct: at heart we're pacific and loving; the fault lies with the social conditions our species has set up for itself? Although I would desperately like to agree with Rousseau on this question, brain research suggests the former alternative. Whenever you interfere with the inhibitory influences of the cerebral hemispheres, something inevitably surfaces that suggests that there's a jungle down there.

Over untold millennia and with great effort, nature has subdued, but not tamed, the wild beasts that reside within the human mind. Those creatures no longer run freely through the psychic plains, but are confined beneath a trap door, upon which is written, "Open at your own risk."

To be fair, the inner space trippers at Mind World are given due warning about possible ogres that may be hiding just below the surface, seething to get out. They sign a statement that says, "A flight to inner space is not recommended for individuals suffering from a major mental illness, such as schizophrenia, manic-depressive disorder, or seizure disorders." Nothing is said about people like myself who, I expect, fit into the category of neurosis—a great, grand diagnosis especially favored by Freud, but one that we don't hear so much about in these freewheeling times. Today concepts such as superego and guilt are treated as curious museum pieces.

After a few minutes on the synchronizer, I yanked off the goggles and earphones. Okay . . . maybe I'm not as concentrated or relaxed or productive as I wish; but at least I have a sense of myself that the synchronizer served only to dispel and disorient. Besides, I'm wondering what it says about ourselves when inner peace and satisfaction are thought to be dependent upon self-centered explorations of one's own mind rather than explorations directed toward the world and other people. Of course introspection is important—I wouldn't be a practicing neuropsychiatrist if I didn't believe that—but mind machines don't bring insights, only psychic isolation and a furtherance of narcissism. Indeed, high-tech voyages toward self-discovery might just provide the most frightening experience of all: buying one of the machines, going home, putting on the goggles and earphones, and finding yourself at home with . . . nobody but yourself.

I'll not be returning to Mind World. After much effort I've established over the years an uneasy coexistence with my inner demons. As a result I'm very wary of anything that gives them a temporary advantage or opportunity to reassert themselves. For the most part the head that arises out of the psychic mire isn't likely to be a friendly one.

I'm sure I could do battle with them and win. It's happened that way from time to time. But right now I'll save twenty-five dollars by sitting back in this chaise lounge, closing my eyes, pointing my face toward the sun, and taking a quiet nap. I've got a feeling that with some luck it will be a tranquil sleep.

o

CONVERSATIONS
WITH TOBY

When I open the front door of my house, my pet African gray parrot, Toby, greets me by name.

My typical reply is: "Yes, Toby . . . and how are you?"

Sometimes (this can't always be depended upon) he responds, "Come here," or "What's up?" or, my particular favorite if it's late in the afternoon, "Open the bar."

Are we communicating? Of course. Are we sharing meaning? In a way, I suppose, we are. I suspect Toby can recognize my footsteps; he usually doesn't call out my name when someone else enters the house. On the whole, though, I am convinced that our communication is not based on Toby's comprehending language. Put another way, our communication is an emotional one, dependent more on the older limbic structures within the brain than on the newer language processing areas within the cerebral hemispheres. This same limbic-cerebral cortex imbalance characterizes the earliest instances of human communication as well.

"Guess what," a three-year-old boy who lives nearby says at the start of each of his sentences. His mother, of course, responds, "What?" At that instant a warm smile breaks out on the child's face. Even at age three he recognizes that his presence has been confirmed, love asserted, connectedness and communication reaffirmed. "Guess what" is often a meaningless phrase in a particular context, but the feelings evoked are far from meaningless. Many social rituals ("How are you?" "I am fine, thank you. How are you?" "I am fine, too.") exist not so much for the communication of information as for emotional sharing: we experience a kind of warmth not unrelated to what's experienced by the little boy when his mother responds with wide-eyed interest, "What?" Being denied that shared warmth can be extremely traumatizing. That's what makes a "cut" or a "snub" so painful, causing our breath to be momentarily taken away, our heart to beat faster. We expected confirmation and approval but met only disdain.

This need for emotional connectedness rather than communication in the strictly linguistic sense impels people to complicate their lives by taking on the care and maintenance of pets. "It's nice to have that warmth and pressure against your body when you're once again forced to sleep alone," a recently divorced woman mentioned to me. Her devoted Saint Bernard provides her with a presence and emotional connectedness she no doubt considers safer and wiser than being with a human companion taken to bed in a desperate attempt to stave off isolation and loneliness.

At the limbic level the warmth and pressure of that dog against my friend's leg corresponds, I suspect, to the interchange between the three-year-old and his mother or the dialogue that I have with Toby as I return home from work. Pets provide emotional "feeding" rather than the opportunity for communication in the traditional sense. And apparently that feeding must be life-sustaining, since the elderly, the housebound, and the lonely with pets do better and often live longer than those without pets. If it's communication, the sharing of information, we want, we speak to each other rather than to pets. Or should.

I arrived at these conclusions about the limbic brain—emotions—pet connection during a conversation with Aaron H. Katcher, a psychiatrist and coauthor of *New Perspectives on Our Lives with Companion Animals*. Katcher and I were coparticipants at an international symposium sponsored by the Smithsonian entitled Man and Beast Revisited. During one of the breaks, we discussed the implications of pet ownership on general health and longevity.

Katcher has observed that talking to pets can lower pet owners' blood pressure and slow their pulse. There are even ritualized ways of talking to pets. When asking questions of their animals, people tend to use low volume, high pitch, a slow rate of speech, and a rising inflection. This is similar to the way parents talk to their infants.

Pet owners also display a typical pattern of facial expression: a faint smile on the pet owner's face; the eyelids lowered or even completely closed; and the jaw tilted slightly forward. "The general appearance of the face suggests relaxation and intimacy," says Katcher.

Relaxation and intimacy involve a diminishing of the influence of the sympathetic nervous system—the arousal network originating in the hypothalamus—coupled with the dominance of the parasympathetic nervous system. This realignment of priorities from "fight or flight" to "relax and smell the flowers" takes place within the limbic areas of the brain and doesn't require either conscious thought or language communication. It's all a matter of visceral reactions, "gut responses" in the brain—pure, unadulterated emotions.

Emotional responsiveness to animals can provide clues about people's future emotional responsiveness to members of their own species. Many children who torture animals turn up years later with the diagnosis of criminal psychopaths. This behavior is part of a triad, consisting of fire setting, bed wetting, and the torture of animals. Torturing pets is the clearest indicator for future failures of socialization, such as sadism and psychopathy. These deteriorations of emotional communication extend over a lifetime.

At the other extreme of limbic responsiveness are those people who seem to get along better with pets and other animals than they do with other people. They don't have to reason with a pet, can maintain complete control over the situation at all times, and can terminate all interaction at a whim—I suspect these issues of control are paramount in the mental lives of such people.

But on occasion the bond between pet owner and pet can also provide a model for continuity and fidelity that in this time of rapid social turnover should give us pause. The example I have in mind concerns an African gray parrot. I think about it whenever someone hears Toby and me talk and then suggests by word or glance that it's perhaps not quite proper, perhaps a little weird, that a brain doctor and a parrot should engage so easily in conversational exchanges.

No, the African gray parrot in question isn't Toby. It's the oldest stuffed bird known to exist, dating back to 1702. It can be seen today in the Norman Undercroft Museum at Westminster Abbey. The bird lived for over forty years with the Duchess of Richmond and Lennox, the woman who sat for the original figure of Britannia used on the coinage. Although we have no record of their conversations, we can suspect that the animal was quite attached to the duchess, for it died within only a few days of its mistress.

Now that's real limbic communication, wouldn't you agree?

RUNNING
ON 10 PERCENT

The question I am most frequently asked about the human brain during my lectures in various parts of the world is: "Do you agree with the claim that we use something like only ten percent of our brain?" Behind that question lies the unstated assumption that we could all achieve genius if we only tried a bit harder. If we could somehow figure out a way to increase our brain's potential, so the reasoning goes, nothing could stop any one of us from becoming another Einstein or Mozart. The idea is appealing in its egalitarian implications, but brain research doesn't provide much support for the concept that we're all potential geniuses.

At UCLA researchers used PET scanning, a procedure employing a radioactively labeled glucose-sugar solution that is injected and then traced to the area of the brain where it is metabolized. These scans help to compare the performance of people who scored very well on IQ tests with that of individuals performing within only an average range. The researchers started off with the seemingly reasonable idea that "smarter brains" work harder, generate more energy, and consume more glucose. Like light bulbs, the brains of "bright" people were expected to illuminate more intensely than those of "dimwits" with a reduced wattage. The results turned out to show just the opposite: those who performed best on the IQ test tended, on average, to produce cooler, more subdued PET scan patterns (blue and green colors), while their less intellectually gifted counterparts lit up like miniature Christmas trees ("hot" red and various oranges hues). The brain of the less-intelligent person seemed to have to work harder to achieve less.

Such biological constraints on human intelligence offend some people, who find it difficult to accept the idea that nature could apportion giftedness the same way as, say, beauty. But autopsies performed on the brains of extraordinarily gifted people demonstrate striking neurological differences from the average. For instance, a now dead artist who possessed a photographic memory as a child and retained it into adulthood was discovered to possess a brain with twice the usual thickness in the area that processes vision (the visual cortex, a cap-shaped area toward the back of the brain). In a person gifted with perfect pitch, it was auditory cortex, the sound reception and analyzing area, that was thicker. And Einstein's brain contained a greater number than usual of glial cells, a network of cells that provide structural and functional support for the brain cells, the neurons.

As far as we can tell, the brains of highly gifted people do not differ solely by having more cells or by being bigger than usual. For one thing, larger brains are associated with larger physiques. Charlemagne, a big man, had a larger brain than Einstein, but he also had a bigger heart, liver, and pancreas. Nor is a huge number of brain cells a distinguishing factor. It's believed more likely that the psychobiological basis for genius may be the number of networks or the intricacy of their interweaving. Brain cells have to be functionally connected into networks so that nerve signals may be widely distributed throughout the brain. A more elaborate and sophisticated network allows greater powers of communication between nerve cells, even cells located vast distances from each other.

Intellectual giftedness, in addition to being associated with the ability to perceive, comprehend, and reason at an extraordinary level, frequently occurs in association with an underlying "quickness" of response. Comedians illustrate this in their routines when they employ double takes to characterize a slow-witted character. Research supports the notion that for smart people, the interval required to make some simple decisions is shortened. For instance, the inspection time required to judge which of two briefly presented lines is the longer correlates strongly with IQ: the shorter the time, the higher the IQ.

Before we decide that not much can be done to improve our mental capacities, consider the encouraging results of intelligence studies. An "enriched environment"—a more challenging cage for rats, more things to do and talk about for humans—enhances the brain's general functioning, making the individual smarter and more challenging and interesting to be around. In rats, neuronal dendrites (nerve cell extensions) are more elaborated. (Picture a tree in January and compare that same tree's appearance in July.) Comparisons of brain cells in humans growing up in enriched versus psychologically impoverished environments haven't been carried out, for obvious ethical and humanitarian reasons. But there is little doubt that a similar process takes place: not more cells or bigger cells, but *increasing numbers* of cell connections, culminating in more elaborate and intricate neuronal networks. In practical terms this means that even in old age we can exert some measure of control over how smart or creative we are. (In the case of brain disease, of course, this tenet doesn't hold.) Our activities, habits, and interests not only define our personalities in the psychological sense, but actually affect the physical structure of our brain. Throughout our lives we can enhance our brain's performance and modify and enrich its structure by extending our range of interests and expanding our intellectual horizons.

In another PET study, also from UCLA, trained musicians were compared with people who had no specialized musical training or interest. The researchers discovered that the trained musicians process music in the left hemisphere—not surprising, since ordinarily the left hemisphere is taken up with analyzing and comparing (Mozart compared with, say, Brahms.) The right hemisphere, in contrast, reacts to music holistically—the basic "I like what I like approach"—which doesn't involve too much analysis. Consistent with this, a study found that musical ingenues favor right hemisphere processing. *Even* more interesting were the changes that took place over time as a person became more involved in the analysis and appreciation of music. The PET scan pattern showed a shift toward left hemisphere processing, as if the brain's organization had been altered in response to new knowledge and attitudes: music had become more than simply something to which you tap your foot or nod your head.

Personally, I'm exhilarated at discovering that we can change how our brain operates. All my life I have been uncomfortable with the thought that perhaps our behavior really *is* conditioned by stimulus response and other behavioral strategies derived from closely observing rats sitting in cages or running through mazes. But it now appears that we can literally change our brain for the better as a result of new interests and the development of new talents. What a marvelous opportunity and awesome responsibility! But we can no longer blame anyone or anything other than ourselves if, because of laziness or disinterest, our brain never develops its full potential. And just what is that potential? Can we all become geniuses if we only try hard enough? Perhaps that's expecting more than nature or nurture is capable of conferring, no matter how much we try. But even if we don't all turn out to be Nobel laureates, it's nice to know that brain research is confirming a long cherished and valued belief: when it comes to our mind and its development, we retain a gratifying measure of control after all.

Perhaps soon the most frequent question I will be asked about the brain will undergo a small but significant change to: "Is it true that we *stimulate* something like only ten percent of our brain?"

And if brain research continues to support and expand its current findings, my answer will be a definite "Yes!"

A TEMPORARY
REPRIEVE

I've never forgotten my first experience with a schizophrenic. Even after twenty years I still remember that tall, well-dressed man of about twenty-two who begged me to do something about his neighbor whose machine was stealing his thoughts. My impulse was to respond reasonably: "What kind of machine? Surely you must know that such things aren't possible?"

How strange and disconcerting it was for me as a doctor of twenty-six to discover that reason is as ineffectual with a schizophrenic as a political harangue delivered to a community of strangers who speak different languages. The schizophrenic's impermeability to logic, reason, discussion, or other "rational" approaches struck a deeply disturbing note at the time. I had been taught all my life that everything could benefit from the application of reason. I mention these considerations as background for evaluating those claims, increasingly frequent nowadays, of a major discovery that explains schizophrenia. But the effort to find one chemical explanation for the illness is a variation on the same mistaken notion. Sometimes the culprit is an errant or truant chemical. Or the disorder may be in the genes. Such a claim was recently made by a British team of psychiatrists who documented the presence of a "susceptibility gene" on chromosome 5 in Icelandic and British families. These "explanations" are always interesting for the promise that they hold out for the future dismantling of influencing machines and the reinstatement of reason to its place as the predominant determinant in the life of the mind.

But for every such discovery, another soon surfaces that contradicts it. The same issue of the journal that reported the susceptibility gene contains a study that failed to show peculiarities of any DNA sequencing in families from northern Sweden containing schizophrenics. Incidentally, such discrepancies bear more on the nature of the illness than on the quality or correctness of the research of these various investigators.

Our knowledge of illnesses, particularly those involving the mind, evolves in a consistent, if not always predictable, pattern. We tend to lump together in one category all those who display a common symptom. For centuries, hearing voices was considered a sign of demonic possession. Later, the interpretation was changed from the theological "possession" to a psychiatric "madness." But not everyone who hears voices suffers from the same illness, any more than all headache sufferers are plagued with migraine. Some do have the same afflictions, of course, but others have brain tumors, abnormalities of the walls of blood vessels within the brain, or stress and strain along the muscles at the base of the neck. Theories about schizophrenia are following similarly diverse paths. It's likely that mutations at different chromosome locations account for why some schizophrenics have abnormalities at one site and others at another site, while the vast majority show no chromosomal disturbances whatsoever. Scientists call this disorder "heterogenous," a ten-dollar word meaning that *many* causes can lead the schizophrenic to believe that his thoughts are controlled by a machine.

More important than the details of the latest "explanation" for schizophrenia is the issue of what attitude the physician should maintain toward patients afflicted with such a disabling and pernicious illness.

At one time my attitude toward such patients was pessimistic and, to be perfectly truthful, somewhat resentful. Caring for such patients was a frustrating experience for me; I wanted to care for patients who were young, verbal, interesting, and likely to get better. And then I met Beth. In a way she cured me of these unphysicianly attitudes, though, I am sad to say, I was never able to cure her.

Beth's diagnosis was chronic undifferentiated schizophrenia, a largely abandoned term that expresses a profound hopelessness about the patient's future. It also reveals the doctor's unwillingness to take the time and trouble to *differentiate* and explore possibilities that might make a difference in the patient's treatment and progress.

Twice a week I sat with Beth. She rarely spoke, and if she did, it was as if she were inviting me to enter into a conversation that went nowhere. At such times I had to force myself to listen and fend off preoccupations of my own. Three or four times a year she would do something sufficiently bizarre and upsetting to others that she would require hospitalization (on one occasion she took off all her clothes and sat on the roof of an apartment building with her feet dangling off the edge).

"What's the point of all this?" I asked my supervisor one Friday afternoon when I could hardly contain my impatience. "Her life is an unending series of hospitalizations, discharges from the hospital for a short period, and then rehospitalizations."

I think of his response now whenever I encounter a patient suffering from a serious neurological or emotional disorder for which there is no cure.

"Not every patient can be cured, but if the doctor can't cure his patient, he can still provide that patient with something incredibly valuable. The doctor can show the patient that her doctor values her, wishes the best for her, in a way *loves* her. Don't undervalue that service, Dr. Restak. Don't be so caught up in rescue fantasies.

"No one—not you, not me, no one—has a right to say that Beth's life isn't meaningful. Even if she has only a month, or a week, or perhaps even just a day of relative freedom from the ravages of her disease, who are you in the grand scheme of things to disparage the value of that temporary reprieve?"

It was a humbling lesson. But I'm glad I learned it when I was still a young doctor. I have benefited from it ever since. And I like to think my patients have benefited as well.

o

THE MIND: MIRROR OF THE BRAIN

What's so special about the brain? A machine can already play chess better than most humans. Given enough time, science will explain how the brain works. Someday scientists will be able to create minds that will have nothing to do with brains. It's only our egocentrism that convinces us that you have to have a brain in order to think."

This statement is fairly typical of what some people now say about the human brain. But even as a person speaks these words, interesting things are going on in his or her brain. For instance, the sentence "What's so special about the brain?" involves a network of neurons, perhaps millions, certainly hundreds of thousands, undulating and pulsing together in what one neuroscientist once described as an "enchanted loom."

Even the most sophisticated model of the mind must involve a modification of the neuronal networks that make up the brain of the person who formulates the model. Additional modification must take place in the brains of those to whom he conveys this marvelous knowledge.

In short, one cannot step outside the "frame" provided by the human brain and say, "Let's just see how things really are, independent of all that neurological stuff." The reason this can't be done? It's very similar to why we can't close our eyes before a mirror and watch ourselves asleep.

No one has ever thought, been inspired, learned, taught, perceived—fill in any human mental process you choose—without using his or her own brain. Indeed, are we anything *other* than our brain? Such a question is a variation on what physicist Edward Harrison, in a marvelous book, *Masks of the Universe*, terms the "containment puzzle."

If anyone claims to have formulated a complete and faithful representation of, say, the universe, then that explanation must contain the cosmologist conceiving and thinking about that universe. This, of course, leads to an infinite regress: the universe contains the cosmologist conceiving the universe that contains the cosmologist conceiving the universe that contains . . . and so on.

Compare this to a person using his brain to conceive what the mind is "really all about" without any reference to the brain. This, too, leads to an infinite regress. The brain's activity formulates a notion about how the mind might exist independent of the brain, perhaps in some computer circuit. But even this idea depends on a representation within the brain of the claim that the mind need not depend on the brain. Within the brain's cortical activity is embedded the thought "What is so special about the brain?"

Brain posits mind, and as it does, networks of active neurons correspond to the representation of what philosophers call "mind." If one alters or dampens that network (perhaps by getting drunk and acting very mindlessly indeed, or falling asleep and thereby assigning all philosophical speculations to the void), mind diminishes or ceases to exist.

Few would argue, I expect, that an individual brain can expect to plumb the depths of its own functioning. Psychoanalysts established decades ago that few of us are the best sources of information about why we think and act the way we do. Brain lesions, too, can leave in their wake disturbances in behavior and perception to which the afflicted individual seems oblivious. For example, a stroke on the right side of the brain is often accompanied by denial that there's anything amiss. On occasion this denial can lead to tragedy, as with one of my patients who sideswiped another car in his left lane minutes after suffering a stroke that had deprived him of leftward vision. Because the brain damage responsible for this visual loss was due to a stroke on the *right* side of my patient's brain, he was oblivious to the objects and events off to his left.

Nor do many brains working together do any better when it comes to self-insight. So far neuroscientists, each concentrating on different brains and different aspects of these brains, have failed to come up with an overall understanding of how the brain works. This should not be surprising, since the insight, however brilliant it might appear, would have to involve the brain of the person who had this insight, as well as the brains of those to whom the insight was communicated.

"Truth," "understanding," "proof," "science," "progress"— each has evolved in tandem with the organization of our brain. If our brain were organized differently, the answer to the "ultimate" questions would be different, or there would be different "ultimate" questions or perhaps no "ultimate" questions at all.

My Pekingese, Bentley, lying at my feet as I write, seems curiously unconcerned about whether he possesses a mind. I know that he has a brain, and I also know that it is organized differently from my own. Neither of us, however, can step outside our brain and stare as through a window at what's going on "outside."

So closely are we intertwined with our brain that to speak of mind without brain is to say nothing at all. Perhaps we should follow Ludwig Wittgenstein's advice: "What one cannot speak about we must pass over in silence."

Of course, he came to that opinion because of the particular way *his* brain operated, his mind worried.

The seeker after knowledge about the brain also encounters another paradox, first mentioned seven hundred years ago by Saint Thomas Aquinas. He said that it's impossible to get to know everything there is to know about anything, even something as simple as a blade of grass.

Our knowledge of the blade of grass, like our knowledge of the brain, depends very much on the kinds of questions that interest us. What is its chemical composition? How does it grow from a seed? How does the individual blade of grass fit into the lawn as a whole? And, come to think of it, why has the blade of grass, along with its companions on my neighbor's lawn, gotten as high as it has?

With the last question, the blade of grass has become intertwined, via my thinking about it, with my neighbor's pesky laziness. Instead of tending to his lawn, providing it with a much needed haircut, he is at the moment no doubt engaged in other pursuits—perhaps sitting on his porch speculating on whether we can ever get to know everything there is to know about the human brain.

Ask certain questions, pursue particular lines of inquiry rather than others, learn a bit more, and then fashion a more sophisticated question; by such maneuvers "everything there is to know" gets defined. And since the limitation on this process is nothing other than the limitations of the human brain, a certain circularity enters into our inquiry.

An inquiring into "everything there is to know" is itself the product of the human brain. Indeed, our search for everything there is to know about the brain would have to include the operation of that very brain that asks, impishly, "Will scientists ever discover everything there is to know about the human brain?"

If I wish to know everything about a blade of grass, I must at some point inquire how it is that a blade of grass could possibly weigh sufficiently in my estimation as to conjure up a sense of resentment toward my neighbor. Why is it that I believe, though he doesn't, that a blade of grass should be so long and no longer, lest the neighborhood suffer a decline?

By means of such inquiries, the blade of grass has penetrated into the biological, aesthetic, psychological, and sociological spheres. And what is the unifying force that makes all of these permutations possible? None other, of course, than the brain that asks these questions—my brain.

It's likely that the blade of grass that so intrigued Aquinas is as unknowable in its basic reality as the brain that inquires into the everything about which it wishes to know.

Blades of grass and brains can be macerated, churned in blenders, and analyzed. Their chemical composition and physiological processes can then be separately investigated. But investigation along one line often precludes another. And at a certain level of structural analysis the system simply ceases to function. For example, if you take away a critical component, neuronal transmission ceases within the brain.

A variation on the "everything there is to know" question is "What is the meaning of the human brain?" To which, I suspect, Saint Thomas might well respond, "What is the meaning of a blade of grass?"

Let me make the point slightly differently.

Over the past six generations members of the community of Oak Bluffs, on Martha's Vineyard, have been holding Illumination Night. Outside and inside tiny gingerbread houses are displayed beautifully decorated silk-skin lanterns that, when lit, provide a stream of multicolored lights.

In recent years visitors to the island have been heard to inquire, "What is the meaning of this?" What facts would we need to know in order to know everything there is to know about it?

The late editor Henry Beetle Hough, writing on Illumination Night, captured the essence of why we can never get to "know everything there is to know" about anything. With Zen-like wisdom he wrote:

> *Illumination began long, long ago in the difference between light and dark. Beyond this, your own explanation must be sufficient unto itself, as good as any. No symbolism was ever officially declared.*
>
> *What may be most comfortably assumed is that the lights kept at night at the original tents long ago increased more and more until the magnificent blooming reached its present proportions all by itself.*
>
> *What it means is what it is.*

THINKING
ABOUT KNOWING

S pring cleaning this year unearthed an unexpected find. My ten-speed bike, long presumed stolen, surfaced in the garage beneath a clutter of boxes and discarded rugs. It had been years. Could I still ride it?

A half hour later I stood with it in the driveway. Hesitantly I mounted and pushed off. Then came an instant of pure terror as I found myself sitting on a seat that seemed much too high, hunched over a handlebar that seemed turned back in the wrong direction. My God! . . . My balance was off. . . . I would surely fall. . . . Was there still time to jump off?

Suddenly something clicked inside my brain. My legs took over and started pumping. At the same instant, I leaned my shoulders forward and balanced myself. After the terror and clumsiness of a moment before, my gracefulness was worthy of the attention of Balanchine himself. I spent the next hour pedaling happily around my neighborhood.

Frankly, I often find myself responding the way I did that day on the bike. I start off thinking that I can't do something simply because I can't verbalize the process. Then I try it and find that I *can* do it. Although I still can't explain how.

The philosopher Gilbert Ryle described this distinction as that between "knowing how" (my retained ability to ride the bicycle) and "knowing that" (my inability to consciously recall and relate the details of how one rides a bicycle). Contemporary psychologists have investigated Ryle's distinction and have discovered that often we know things we don't even know that we know.

Imagine a situation in which the letters in this sentence are inverted. After some practice you'd be able to decipher the words. With additional practice you'd get better at it and faster. Most interesting of all, your performance would improve independently of your ability to remember its contents or even that you had ever seen the sentence before. Information is first analyzed at the level of visual pattern. Then meaning is given to the pattern. Only then does comprehension follow.

Next imagine yourself in yet another study: You are presented with a list of words not altered in any way and asked to memorize the list. Long after you have forgotten the list you will learn that same list much faster than originally. And yet, mysteriously, you might never recall having seen those words before. Who learned the list? "Why, I did, of course, and very efficiently, too," you may respond. But then answer this: Why is it that even though your superior performance the second time around proves acquaintance with the words, you don't recall previously encountering them? How can you remember if you can't recall?

Those who are philosophically inclined may wish to ponder how it is that we can learn without knowing that we have learned.

Consider one last example, this time from a neurologist's practice. A patient who has suffered a stroke may find himself unable to identify other people from their facial appearance. He may recognize them by the sound of their voice, but facial features alone fail to elicit a response.

Now show such a patient pictures of friends and relatives intermixed with pictures of complete strangers. While verbally the patient gives no more sign of recognizing familiar faces than he does of recognizing unfamiliar ones, nonverbally he exhibits signs of recognition of the familiar faces. Tests aimed at measuring electrical skin conductance demonstrate that recognition is taking place at the level of the autonomic nervous system. Literally, the patient fails to come up with a name and fails at conscious recognition, and yet his skin conductance response clearly indicates recognition has taken place at a nonverbal level. As explained by the experimenters, Daniel Tranel and Antonio Damasio, this curious phenomenon indicates "that the knowledge on which recall or recognition depends is laid down at different levels of the central nervous system, some of which are inaccessible to consciousness."

Such findings among normal people and the neurologically impaired contrast with the past two thousand years of Aristotelianism, which states that "a thing cannot both be and not be at the same time." In the world outside the philosopher's study, we understand it can be both raining and not raining at the same time and, to some extent, at the same place, as we see in sun showers. We can also know something (how to ride a bike), not know that we know it (my momentary terror when astride the ten-speed monster), and not be able to explain to anyone else exactly what it is that we know.

Perception, recognition, memory—all three processes are embedded within the brain via a hierarchical scheme. Failure at the highest level (conscious awareness—"knowing that one knows") doesn't mean the absence of knowledge.

One of the impediments to self-understanding, it seems to me, is our insistence that "real knowledge" involve our capacity to bring our knowledge into conscious awareness. Modern brain research, on the other hand, suggests that knowledge involves dynamic, evolving patterns that are stored at multiple levels in the nervous system. This exciting, scary insight explains such things as intuition, hunches, reading other people's intentions by observing their body language, and so on.

We all know more than we can say. Recognition of this fact demands a flexibility in our responses, a willingness to "let go" and permit what knowledge we may possess to express itself without the chattering interference of conscious awareness. After all, that's the way I learned to ride a bike all over again.

THOSE EYES

E very morning at seven o'clock, just moments after getting out of bed and an hour and a half before heading out to work, a father sits at the bedside of his son, Scotty, who has been in a coma for seven years. At age seventeen Scotty was hit by a truck while bicycling in preparation for a competitive race; he has never recovered from that head injury. Since the accident, Scotty has never spoken, but his eyes are often open, and he can move those eyes to follow his father's movements in the room. His father says that Scotty is somehow dimly conscious of the events going on around him.

Two years ago Scotty was returned to Georgetown University Hospital to undergo tests to determine whether, as his father claimed, this young man could respond—partially, primitively—to events around him. Or whether, as the doctors claimed, Scotty was only reacting on a brain stem level, without any real awareness of himself and the world.

Far below the cerebral cortex and limbic system, those areas largely responsible for our thoughts and emotions, lies the brain stem. This area, which includes the midbrain, pons, and medulla, carries out more humble but vital tasks, such as maintaining blood pressure, regulating our pulse and breathing, and, most important from the mental point of view, keeping us awake. A stroke or a blood clot in the brain stem can, as with the late Karen Ann

Quinlan, render a person deeply and permanently unconscious. In most instances this unconsciousness is obvious to both doctors and relatives. But occasionally nature plays a cruel jest. Certain patients may periodically open their eyes, appearing to look around the room and make eye contact with those standing at the bedside. The patient may even appear to cry, wince in pain, or move as if stretching or assuming a more comfortable position. But the appearance of alertness and intention is deceptive. All of these behaviors can be carried out as an automatic reflex mechanism originating in the brain stem despite the patient's deep and irreversible coma. The technical term for the condition is "coma vigil," and, as with Scotty, it can create false hopes in relatives, along with puzzlement and confusion among doctors not familiar with the condition.

Modern medical technology has made situations like Scotty's possible. Improved ambulance and emergency services, CAT scans, prompt neurosurgical operations, sophisticated intensive care regimens: thanks to these advances, Scotty and perhaps hundreds of others like him now exist in a limbo, not quite dead, but not fully alive, either.

At the other end of the spectrum, it's a curious but undeniable fact that a person can appear completely unconscious and yet be at least partially receptive to events in the surrounding environment. (That is one of the reasons surgeons and others present at operations do not offer prognostications, particularly unfavorable ones, while within earshot of the anesthetized patient.) Scotty, in contrast, appears to be awake, but actually is in a state of profound unconsciousness. He can move his eyes toward the source of a sound or blink whenever someone pretends to push a finger or an instrument toward his eyes. On occasion these responses even appear specific to the stimulus. For instance, Scotty will turn his eyes in the direction of his father's voice if his father approaches the bed. Such behaviors often bring a patient's relatives into conflict with the doctors. "How could he turn his eyes toward me?" seems a sensible question—unless one knows that this seemingly prescient decision can be carried out at the brain stem level. It was in order to resolve just such a disagreement that Scotty was brought to Georgetown University Hospital.

The tests began. Lights flashed into Scotty's open eyes created activity in the visual cortex of the back of the brain. Beeps and clicks funneled into his ear could be recorded along the auditory pathways from the ear upward through the brain stem. Little in the way of registration occurred, however, within the temporal lobes, where the richness of life's auditory experience—Beethoven's Ninth, for instance—is processed.

The test results revealed, in the neurologist's words, that "the cerebral hemispheres are cut off from the lower brain stem"; nevertheless, Scotty exhibited indications of an altering response to his father's voice, but to nothing else. Is Scotty aware, therefore, of the events going on around him? Certainly not in the way that most people employ the word *aware;* yet Scotty isn't completely oblivious to his surroundings, either.

Many doctors who care for patients like Scotty, myself included, have great difficulty achieving a comfortable attitude toward their charges. For some, any evidence of the patient's partial awareness is something they choose to ignore. Others are vaguely haunted and frightened by the prospect; phrases like the *living dead* or *zombie-like* flit in and out of their consciousness and their conversations. Part of the reason for the difficulty stems, I believe, from the unreasonably preeminent respect we accord to logic, rationality, and communication. We insist that all minds, if they are truly functioning, think, remember, and judge, among other abilities. Most of all, minds must communicate with other minds in ways that don't pose any doubt. But Scotty's communications, particularly those to his father, are of an order of magnitude that makes us uncomfortable. If this is communication, then it is as subtle as the play of sunlight on droplets of rainwater as they roll along the surface of a leaf.

As an additional problem, patients like Scotty don't conform to our insistence that lives always be meaningful. Lying in bed unable to move, speak, or communicate except in patterns that even the experts can't agree really exist—certainly this isn't most people's idea of a "meaningful human life." Yet I have observed for myself that Scotty's pupils dilate and contract and that sweat pours from his forehead whenever his father leans over the bed, looks straight into his face, and speaks very slowly and with an enormous degree of compassion and tenderness. On occasion I have been compelled to leave the room lest I show more emotion than would be appropriate in someone who must help that man make an "objective" decision about what should be done for his son.

We both know that at some point an infection will develop that, unless antibiotics are administered, will prove fatal. At that time, I believe, my place will be to advise against their administration and deliver this devoted father from his ordeal. Scotty's father has already sacrificed a huge chunk of his own life. He is with Scotty or talking about Scotty or thinking about Scotty every waking moment. Some of his friends and family members say that he has become obsessed with his son's tragedy. One of the most painful consequences of Scotty's predicament and his father's response to it was the breakup of the twenty-five-year marriage of Scotty's parents. His mother painfully concluded that Scotty would never recover and that the rest of the family should get back to creating lives for themselves. Scotty's father disagreed. He still hopes for what I believe is impossible: Scotty's recovery.

When Scotty does come down with an infection, I hope to be able to persuade his father that we should not use antibiotics—that, in essence, we should let Scotty die. Such a decision will be extremely difficult for both of us.

It's those *eyes* that mock any attempt by me or anybody else to be absolutely, positively sure that Scotty (if he is in some form of primitive contact with us) would prefer death. It is my fervent hope that at the end, for the sake of all three of us, those eyes will be closed.

WHEN WORDS TRIGGER AN EMOTIONAL RESPONSE

H ave you ever noticed that some people become slightly unglued—and sometimes a good deal more—whenever they hear certain words? *Tax audit, welfare, abortion, mistress, racial quotas*—merely mentioning them can produce marked alterations in personality. A person may stammer, blanch or go red in the face, turn argumentative, and undergo erratic changes in blood pressure and pulse, all in response to a mere word. It's as if the offending term produced a kind of emotional short circuit.

Neuroscientists in recent years have formulated an explanation for what happens in the brain during these word-induced emotional short circuits.

The amygdala, a small almond-shaped nucleus within the limbic system of the brain, selects and ties together the varied experiences that make up our lives. Because of the amygdala, some of the stimuli that bombard us every second are imbued with positive or negative emotions. They are then encoded in our brain, where they provide underpinnings for memory and personality.

Usually the emotional flavor imparted by the amygdala is hardly noticeable. It also varies between people. If you had a happy childhood, words like *family* and *marriage* have a slight but definitely pleasant tinge. If your childhood was unhappy, the same words have a slightly negative effect.

On the basis of the subtle and sometimes not-so-subtle impact of certain words, each person literally lives in his or her own reality. Two people may have dinner together on Valentine's Day but be emotionally light-years apart. The word *love*, for example, can arouse feelings of claustrophobia in one listener. In another the word *love* triggers feelings of affection, commitment, or solace. Because the same word has different associations, people respond to it differently.

In the brain neuronal networks involving the limbic system have endowed words such as *love* with positive or negative emotional coloring, depending on a person's life experiences.

With practice, I've discovered, it's possible to learn to detect the emotional coloration your amygdala has given to certain words. But you have to be quick about it. Within a split second of hearing a word or phrase, try to detect the first subtle glimmer of feeling.

Psychoanalysis, Zen, and certain forms of meditation are directed at early detection of evanescent interior feelings that determine so much of what we do and accomplish in our lives. In order to "know thyself," it's necessary to detect these first glimmers of feeling. This process of automatic emotional response to words becomes more established the longer we live, partly explaining why the old are more inflexible than the young. What happens at the level of the brain? It's likely that neuronal networks within the cortex (particularly the frontal and prefrontal areas, where concepts and symbols are elaborated) are linked with reverberating networks within the "emotional brain" (the limbic system). Each time these networks fire, it becomes easier for the circuits to be reactivated. That's how habits are formed.

But all of this can be changed if we can only learn early on to detect and control our tendency to overreact at the mention of a specific word or term. It's also an example of the exciting ways that brain research can contribute to our effort to understand ourselves. To do that, we must ultimately understand our brain and how it works because, in the final analysis, we *are* our brain.

Moreover, the partitions that philosophers and psychologists have set up in the past (thinking, emotions, memory, etc.) are highly artificial. The brain simply isn't organized that way at all.

Says Peter Gloor of the Montreal Neurological Institute, "We experience these phenomena as unified events. It is therefore not too unlikely that somewhere in the brain the contributions of the various areas involved in the elaboration of the components of these experiential mechanisms coalesce."

Someday, I believe, these neuroscientific insights may be applied in areas far removed from science as we presently understand it. Words, for instance, may no longer have the power to short-circuit rationality, cooperation, and communication. For instance, take the way words are sometimes used as weapons.

"I think I'll jam Tom's circuits by suggesting he's a reactionary," thinks Phil. "That always gets a rise out of him. That'll end the argument."

But if Tom has learned to control his emotional responsiveness to being called a reactionary, the game is over. The two adversaries have no choice but to deal with the real issues and not simply one person's tendency to blow a fuse in response to another's vocabulary.

And imagine the benefits that could ensue if the delegates at the United Nations could learn to identify their emotional overreaction to words such as *détente, human rights violations, apartheid, terrorism.*

The development of such capacities within our leaders could turn out to be cost-effective. With luck we might even be able to save ourselves the expense of a couple of F-15s. Or even a war or two.

LOOKING
INTO THE WINDOWS
OF THE SOUL

A jade dealer in San Francisco a decade ago seemed to possess a remarkable power. After displaying a tray of rare pieces, he was able to discern at a glance which item the customer found most appealing. Then, just seconds before the customer spoke, the dealer raised the price of that single item: "Everything on the tray is a thousand dollars . . . except for *this*, which is fifteen hundred."

One day a customer from Los Angeles came into the store wearing dark glasses and indicated his choice before the dealer could say a word about price. The store manager was convinced the dealer's remarkable intuitive powers had suddenly failed him. What was the problem? What had happened to the dealer's sixth sense?

The jade dealer had mastered the art of observing the tiny expansion of the pupil of the eye that accompanies interest and excitement. While ostensibly studying the tray of jade, the dealer would actually observe his customers' eyes. This time the dark glasses had deprived the dealer of his advantage.

With a little practice anyone can acquire the skill of reading pupils, but pupillary changes provide only a small portion of the information conveyed by the eye. Eye contact is equally revealing. When two people look each other in the eye, the strength and intensity of their mutual gaze provides a measure of their interest.

But the meaning of that prolonged eye contact depends very much on the social situation.

Most of us look longer at people and things we like, more briefly at objects of our disapproval. For lovers, lengthy and intense eye contact is a special form of intimacy. The lover looks at—indeed, stares at—his beloved, who interprets this as a sign of affection. The pupils also dilate. In some parts of the world, women still put drops of belladonna ("beautiful lady") in their eyes to dilate the pupils artificially and thereby enhance attractiveness.

Change the social situation, and a prolonged gaze may shift in meaning from love toward dislike or even hatred. Martial artists never lower their eyes in the midst of an encounter. Good poker players know the value of an intense, cold, analytic stare. And if you have ever been cross-examined in court, you know an interrogator's unflinching eye contact can rattle you.

Centuries ago some romantic referred to the eyes as the "windows of the soul," no doubt referring to the eyes' expressive power. Eyes can express agreement, as when we "see eye to eye" with someone during a discussion. Or the eyes can express possible deceit, as when one "can't look us in the eye." The eyes can also express humility. The eyes are cast down whenever one enters a sanctuary of one of the world's great religions. And nuns and monks during the Middle Ages were admonished for their lack of humility if they gazed too intently into their superior's eyes or into the eyes of one another.

But a certain amount of eye contact is necessary to assure us of our own existence. Not to be seen is not to be acknowledged, not to exist. Few things are more irritating than a clerk's telegraphing his hostility by not responding to our attempt to catch his eye. Yet if we express our displeasure too directly, he may look us "straight in the eye" and try to "stare us down." If we're superstitious, we might even fear that he will give us the "evil eye."

Comfortable amounts of eye contact vary enormously. The entertainer can't get enough. Women generally make more eye contact than men, children and adults more than adolescents, extroverts more than introverts. Autistic people rarely, if ever, make eye contact, and schizophrenics share gazes with few except other schizophrenics. Depressives turn their gaze downward. Among neurotics there doesn't seem to be a reliable pattern; some avoid others' eyes, and some stare rudely.

We usually look directly at others twice as much while listening as when talking. When we start a sentence, we tend to look away, probably to avoid being distracted from what we want to say. When we listen and look, we miss fewer words and respond to the non-verbal components of what's said. Pompous people look as much when speaking as when listening, perhaps because they feel that what the other person says is comparatively unimportant. The message a sustained gaze conveys while talking is: "You listen to me. What I have to say is more important than your babbling."

Most of us, perhaps mercifully, remain largely unaware that our eyes reveal so much information about us. Those who are aware tend, like the jade-buying customer from Los Angeles, to prefer dark glasses. A pair of "shades" identifies the "cool cat," a reference to the communicative power of the cat's pupils, which dilate when the animal is excited. Wearing a pair of shades, the cool cat can study other people's emotions while keeping his own responses hidden. Torturers and terrorists are also aware of this. Idi Amin and his followers favored reflective sunglasses. That way the victim not only was deprived of seeing his inquisitor's emotions, but had to gaze at his own terror reflected in the mirrored lenses.

The eye also tells a lot about our physical health. When the doctor, with the help of an ophthalmoscope, looks deep into our eye, he is looking at the optic nerve, the only extension of the brain that can be directly visualized. And on occasion the first sign of a brain tumor is a swelling of the optic nerve as it leaves the brain on its way to the back of the eye. Other brain diseases—multiple sclerosis, for example—are sometimes detectable by a subtle change in the color of the optic nerve.

Observing the eye and speculating about our observations can be fascinating. But we must not be careless in our observations. I learned this during a conversation twenty years ago with a woman in dark glasses. I speculated out loud about why she would be wearing them in a small midtown bar at eleven at night. When I finished, she took my hand in hers, moved it down, and placed it firmly on . . . the head of her guide dog.

o

OUR OWN WORLDS

D ay after day I sit in my consulting room and listen to
those who come to me for help. This is one of my life's
most important structures. My troubled patients have
constructed a life structure, too. They come for my help
because that structure pains, confines, or terrifies them. Structures
can promise release or restraint, and each can present its own
problems. Here are two examples chosen from many:

I once treated a man on a psychiatric ward who scoured the city in
search of discarded mattresses. After dragging or hauling these
veterans of love trysts and night terrors back to his apartment, he
twisted the springs into an intricate floor-to-ceiling tangle. And at
the top of it, off in one corner of the room, he lived his spiderlike
existence.

When the police were called in by the landlord, they stared
dumbfounded for several minutes at this edifice of mattress innards. Finally they did what they thought best. They ripped out the
springs, cut through the network with wire cutters, extracted the
man, and took him to the nearest mental hospital. But not before
they took pictures of his peculiar, steel-wired kingdom, which had
so unsettled their composure.

The man never confided to me what had stimulated him to undertake his vast project. Whenever the subject was brought up, he

became silent. Later I learned that the artist Marcel Duchamp had once constructed something similar, but on a more modest scale:

> *Little pieces of rubber of various sizes and colors that I fastened to the ceiling. They were mostly little bits of rubber bathing caps, which I cut up and glued in place, and which had no particular shape. At the bottom of each piece there was a thick rope, and these were tied to the four corners of the room, so that when you entered the room you couldn't move around because these ropes blocked your way.*

Constructing a prison, whether of wire or rubber, could be viewed as insane, ludicrous, artful, eccentric, or meaningless—depending on the circumstances. But think of it as creating a world in which everything is connected to everything else. Every time that obsessed man changed his position, he set off a tremor that extended to every nook and cranny of this world he had constructed. The most mundane motion thus took on a significance that perhaps the man's actions in the larger world failed to provide him with.

In Duchamp's case the purpose seems to have been slightly different (I've never discovered his explanation). He divided unity, a room, into continents, islands, continental divides, archipelagoes. To travel from one part of his world to another, one had to endure hardships of various kinds. Any explanation beyond that is pure conjecture. Like my patient, Duchamp largely kept to himself the purpose of the world he had made.

Now let me tell you of a fantasy world that occurred to me, inspired by my desire to understand my patient the collector of bedsprings. I'd build a labyrinth of books, not set on shelves, but stacked six or eight feet high with little passageways leading from one area to another.

Here's the plan and purpose that occurred to me within my fantasy. Imagine opening the door to my room, and all you can see are books piled in a wood-supported labyrinth. To enter, you have to hunch down on your knees and begin crawling along a book-lined passageway. There are twists and turns and little islands where you can come off your knees and sit in an enclave about five feet high. There is a lamp there, and you can sit and read with absolutely no one to bother you. You might try, say, the philosophy section. After a while, when you've tired of philosophy, you decide to move along the passageway to literature. You have a passage map to guide you through various routes to the sections that interest you.

No one can disturb you within this specially constructed library. No one standing at the door could determine exactly where you were. You are totally isolated, enjoying complete peace and comfort in the confines of a world totally of your own making.

Imagine that on a typical day you return from the frustrations of your office to this room to spend endless hours reading Plato or Margaret Mead or, in another part of the room, Louis L'Amour. Doesn't this possibility fill you with intense satisfaction? To be alone and perfectly free within one's own world, isolated from noise and pollution and raised voices. What could be more pleasurable? I ask you.

Now imagine that one day you hear voices at the door of your library. You can't see who's speaking, and they can't see you. But hiding in your labyrinth, you're soon certain that they're talking about you. What's worse, they begin to suggest in insulting terms that your paradise of a room is the work of a madman. Imagine, if you can, your feelings if you heard these interlopers knocking your artfully constructed world to the floor, turning your carefully planned labyrinth into chaos.

Would you try to explain to these rude people what the world you constructed meant to you? I suspect not. You would probably spend the days of your consignment in the psychiatric ward planning how you might construct that world all over again when you were freed.

Springs or bits of bathing caps or books—the materials may differ according to time, place, education, perhaps even karma. But ultimately, don't they all serve a common purpose—to make us powerful, godlike; to enable us to create our own perfect, private world?

And when that Eden is destroyed, as it was with my patient, what could possibly be a more appropriate response than silent, sullen resentment?

"When he's with me, everything seems to fall into place. Each moment of the day there is something to do, a structure by which I can define myself. But I really must protect my freedom. I guess what I really want is a man who will love me but spends a lot of time away from the house. That way I can still remain free to do what I want."

The speaker is a woman in her mid-thirties. She pauses and looks at me, hoping I will offer explanation and solution for her problem. But what does a neuropsychiatrist say to a person struggling between the world as she would like it to be and the world as it is?

Without this man her life is a chaos of waking up in strange rooms to the smell of stale cigarettes, irregular hours, sessions before the mirror looking for wrinkles, and worries about venereal infections and cancer. She readily admits that she merely reacts to the events in her life—the backwash of failures to anticipate, plan, organize.

But when she's with him, she feels vaguely confined, as if wearing a dress a size too small that she likes too much to exchange for one the correct size but less flattering.

In my notebook I write: "She is caught in the dilemma between the need for perceived freedom and the need to be embedded in a structure that, it seems, she cannot fashion for herself."

"Do you think it likely he would accept this arrangement whereby you commit to him but you still retain your freedom to do as you like?" I inquire.

. . . A pause . . . Her eyes drop like two loose pearls toward her lap. "No, I don't think so."

"So what will you do if he asks you to marry him?" The question remains suspended in the air like an icicle.

"I'm not sure. . . . One part of me says, 'Go for it. Try it.' The other part says, 'You know it can't work.' "

A psychiatrist faces his own painful and testing identity crisis in moments like these. Should I express by word or gesture my opinion that without this man, or someone like him, her life will likely remain chaotic? Or should I maintain the neutrality that has enabled me to achieve insights about her that, perhaps later, I can use to further advance her self-understanding?

"My job is to help you understand yourself. Once that is achieved, you will be free to decide on your own about how to live your life"—that is more or less the statement I make many times during the course of a patient's treatment.

This patient already understands her need-for-structure versus need-for-freedom dilemma. But understanding hasn't helped; she remains frozen and immobile in the winter landscape of her despair.

What is most important for psychological well-being: freedom to know or freedom to act?

As this unhappy woman and I talk together, street people outside the office hold paper cups as they beg for coins. Some talk to themselves, see visions, hear voices. In earlier and simpler times they would have been in hospitals and eligible for treatment that might help them. But today we've released them to the "freedom" of the streets.

"In doing this, you have not given the severely mentally ill civil liberty. You have merely given them the right to be slaves to their own devastating and debilitating brain disease," said the mother of a mentally ill young woman, who was about the age of the patient sitting before me.

My patient isn't suffering from anything as extreme as the psychosis of some of those outside, but her situation also represents a distortion of what people have traditionally meant when they've spoken about freedom. She has little to do with her family because she feels they limit her "development." She disdains moral and ethical precepts as inhibiting and repressive. She belongs to no organization or group, has no close friends, has made no lasting commitments of any kind, and suffers periodic crises of identity. She talks about supporting the interests of women, minorities, and the oppressed—those most deprived of their freedom—but makes no effort to help the members of any of these groups.

When passing the street people outside the office, she probably wouldn't notice their presence because of her preoccupation with her own thoughts and fantasies. Or if one of them succeeded in attracting her attention, her eyes would almost certainly glaze over to resemble those of a mannequin in the window of one of the department stores where she spends much time.

Wherever and whenever possible she repeats like mantras those phrases that are most important in her life: "internal growth," "self-development," "the person I really am," "the freedom to be me."

As the holidays approach, I expect my patient's difficulties and unhappiness to worsen. She will have to force herself to go among strangers—her parents and her sister. They know very little about her life, and she suspects, not unreasonably, that they would not approve of it if they did. Is it their fault or hers that her family never can keep up with her personality transformations?

"The sadness of a secret life, among others, is not so much that reality is painful as that it has a weaker being, like some image turned on when we wake and turned off when we sleep," according to writer Robert Grudin in *Time and the Art of Living*.

My patient makes me feel guilty, for when I am with her, I am conscious of being a member of a generation that has gotten it all wrong about freedom. In our haste to be free, we've achieved only a petty, self-centered isolation. *Society* has become nothing more than a word we equate with everyone whose interests compete with our own.

And what has this freedom contributed to intimacy? Love is

never having to say you're sorry. Do your own thing. Are you HIV-negative? Who will bring the condoms? "The narcissist has sacrificed the joy of human connectedness for superficial manipulative relationships," as one psychiatrist phrased it during a recent lunch table conversation.

This lack of authentic human connectedness takes individual and collective forms. My patient is convinced that her self-absorption is a form of freedom instead, as I see it, of a limiting, enslaving isolation.

As a society we rail at the sight of street people—blaming the government for not doing more. We avoid accepting the consequences of our misguided attitude toward the freedom and civil rights of mental patients. It is our attitude that consigns these unfortunates to the streets rather than to mental hospitals, where they have a chance of being helped.

Freedom in our age has, indeed, become just another word for nothing left to lose. But there's always more to lose. Every day in innumerable ways my patient becomes less accessible, more entrenched in destructive and alienating patterns of behavior. Indeed, she has surrendered her freedom and has become a slave of her unrestrained self-absorption.

What can I do to understand her and better help her to understand herself? At the same moment I ask myself that question, she looks toward me, expecting some response on my part. As our eyes meet, I turn away from her gaze and become momentarily flustered, for just now I have no answer for her. I ask myself if there is any explanation. Could *any* psychological theory explain this woman and her life? I look at my watch; the hour is up. I am relieved. I'm uncomfortable not having answers that I know are expected of me.

But as she rises to leave, an answer comes to me. A quotation from Goethe. "Do not, I beg of you, look for anything behind phenomena. They are themselves their own lessons."

o

A TREE
THAT TAMES
THE MIND

My brother and sister bought me a bonsai this Christmas. My gratitude was immediately tempered by two considerations: How do I care for this miniature tree, known to me only from scenes out of *The Karate Kid*? And what good is it, what can I do with it?

The first question was easily answered. An expert told me about watering; whether the tree should be inside or outside; how big it should get; when to trim, replant, and so on. The answer to the second question took a little more time.

My bonsai is a shinipaku juniper. More than twenty years old, it looks as if it's been sitting for all of those years on some mountain, fighting off the determined efforts of the wind to permanently dislodge it. Its trunk is gnarled and shaped into a pattern that extends directly horizontal for the first few inches. Then it twists at an almost ninety-degree angle to ascend in a spiral toward the sky.

"Just look at the tree. . . . Be with it. . . . Spend a few minutes every day studying its shape. . . . Interesting things will start to happen," an Oriental friend said when I told her about the tree. She is right. Thanks to this tree, I have relearned something that in my hyperactivity and hypomania I had long forgotten: the pleasure of concentrated attention, the pure joy of escaping distractions and focusing my mind.

Years ago in the Orient children were taught exercises in mental visualization. They sat before a bonsai tree, kept looking at it, finally closed their eyes and visualized the tree's pattern. When they were certain that they had captured the tree in their mental image, they opened their eyes and compared the tree in their mind's eye with the tree sitting right there before them. Along with improving their powers of observation and mental imagery, this exercise helped them to learn the art of sitting still and quieting the "monkey mind." This apt term, originating in India, describes those occasions when ideas and thoughts chaotically leap about in the mind like a monkey swinging through tree branches.

Today that sort of visualization exercise is done only by people who practice meditation, which, unfortunately, gives it a bad name in circles where mental concentration is measured in nanoseconds before distraction sets in.

Psychiatrists rarely mention distraction when they talk about emotional illnesses and disturbances. Yet it is perhaps the most prominent mental disorder of our time.

Whether it's as a result of a fast-paced life-style, television, narcissism, taking on multiple roles, the disintegration of family and community units, or (insert your own favorite here), most people can't sit still or think about only one thing at a time for very long. Monkey mind is epidemic.

Contrast this modern "madness" with Isaac Newton's response when he was asked how he had been able to discover his mechanical system for the universe: *"Nocte dieque incubando"* (By thinking about it day and night).

A similar emphasis on concentration is traditional in the arts, too. There was a portrait at a Paolo Veronese exhibition held at the National Gallery in Washington called *The Dream of St. Helen.* An attractive, elegant, but rather unsaintly-looking woman sits in a high-backed chair, wearing her state robes and bejeweled crown. Her left arm is on an armrest, while her head presses gently against her upturned hand. The exhibition's guidebook states: "Paolo conjures up a somnolent grayed late afternoon light in which one can virtually hear a buzz of silence." But, of course, you can't see or hear much of anything if you can't stand before the portrait for more than fifteen seconds before the urge to move on becomes as peremptory as the itch of poison ivy. Monkey mind at work.

In today's society athletes are the most conspicuous examples of concentrated attention. Even when they're not competing, athletes take a focused, concentrated approach to sport. They look at videotapes for the purpose of storing images or constructing internal models of peak performance. Mental visualization exercises are performed wherein athletes see themselves in their "mind's eye" as winners. These efforts permit athletes to persist, endure, and triumph. "A winner never quits, and a quitter never wins" expresses the value of focused attention combined with persistence.

Similar rules apply within the medical field. "The two most important qualities for a neurosurgeon are honesty and durability," senior neurosurgeon Stacey Rollins recently told me. Durability, of course, is only a synonym for endurance, concentration, and determination.

In the intellectual sphere Freud and Darwin are the best exemplars of the value of holding on to an idea with concentrated tenacity. Like Newton, they thought and brooded and mused until their fundamental theories—of the unconscious and evolution, respectively—became so clear to them that they couldn't imagine how the world could be explained any other way.

Sometimes, though, like now, concentration must be courted on its own merits and without any hope for immediate results.

And so I stare at my bonsai, memorizing its outlines, then closing my eyes and storing a mental image to be compared moments later with the singularity of that tiny tree. In performing this exercise in mental gymnastics, I am confident it will prove helpful sometime in the future.

When we are tired, depressed, overworked, or "hung over," concentration seems impossible. The task is left undone, the enterprise abandoned. For such moments I believe I have the answer to the question "What good is that tree?" It's good for staring at, concentrating, focusing, taming the "monkey mind."

o

TRUTH, JUSTICE, AND THE BRAIN

If a group's familiarity with science correlated with its means of transportation, lawyers and judges would be riding around in buckboards.

Over the past two decades behavioral scientists have made discoveries that bear directly on issues relevant to the courtroom. But for the most part, the judges and lawyers haven't been listening.

Consider the methods commonly employed to interrogate a witness. Research on "eyewitness testimony" reveals that how a question is phrased is very important.

"Did you see the green sports car run the red light and collide with the station wagon?" the witness is asked. A witness who can't remember that there was a stop sign and *not* a traffic signal at the intersection will not be able to offer valid and valuable testimony. In the language of the courtroom, the witness's credibility will be called into question.

A similar loss of credibility can be evoked by deliberately provoking anxiety, anger, or fear in a witness. "Whoever can be aroused either to fear or anger . . . is more easily led to accept the desired pattern of 'cooperation,' even though this may violate his normal judgment," writes psychiatrist William Sargant, an expert on brainwashing.

Despite the findings of Sargant and others, courtroom proceedings, particularly cross-examinations, are routinely conducted in ways that provoke the very emotions that are least likely to result in unbiased testimony by a witness.

"Every accused person has a right to confront his accusers," attorneys routinely respond. Part of this confrontation, they assure us, involves testing whether the witness's testimony can stand up under the pressure of a rigorous cross-examination.

Even granting this point, research on the effects of stress on witness testimony suggests that justice would be better served if efforts were made to decrease the psychological pressures on witnesses. Among the tactics that should be excluded from the courtroom are remarks aimed at disturbing the psychological balance of the witness, sarcasm, deprecatory gestures, and questions that are intentionally complex or ambiguous.

These suggestions are unlikely to be adopted by the court any time soon. Why? Because most lawyers remain convinced, despite scientific evidence to the contrary, that the truth is more likely to be elicited if the witness is subjected to psychological stress.

But the fact is behavioral scientists have discovered that most people—psychopaths and hardened criminals excepted—begin to unravel in direct proportion to the amount of psychological stress inflicted on them. Furthermore, their ability to bear up under the rigors of deliberately inflicted emotional trauma has nothing to do with the truth or falsity of their testimony.

The nature of testimony is another favorite assumption from the horse and buggy era that, unfortunately, enjoys favor among judges and attorneys.

Tremendous emphasis is placed in the courtroom on what a witness says, to the exclusion of *how* it is said. The inflections, accents, pauses, tones, and other subtle nuances of speech can often reveal as much as the words themselves.

Reliance on such "subjective data" in reaching conclusions is suspect, even actively prohibited, in the courtroom. "You must base your conclusions only on the facts of this case and leave your personal feelings out of it," I heard one judge instruct the jury.

Research on the human brain indicates that such instructions not only are unrealistic but place an insuperable burden on a juror. The right hemisphere of our brain specializes in detecting discrepancies between what someone says and how it is said. Listening with the "third ear" is something that we do all the time. We achieve an accuracy of about 80 percent when it comes to correctly identifying and interpreting another person's emotions and motivations.

But with our present system of justice's emphasis on a defendant's Fifth Amendment rights, the jury is deprived of the opportunity of listening with the third ear to the nuances of the defendant's speech. As important as the question "What is he saying in response to the charges against him?" are the questions "How is he saying it?" and "Does he sound like a person who is telling the truth?"

Of course, I'm not suggesting that such a determination should be the sole basis of a juror's decision about "credibility." But I am convinced that denying a juror the opportunity of evaluating the emotional and psychological subtext of a defendant's testimony deprives that juror of a potentially valuable source of information.

Our brain is constructed so as to balance what a person says (coded in the left hemisphere) with how he or she actually says it (a right hemisphere process). To be truly effective, the legal system should model itself on how our brain actually works when we decide about something.

Judicial orders notwithstanding, human beings are not logic machines. Words are an important part of human communication, but they're not the whole story by any means. Perhaps the following should really be a judge's instructions to a jury:

"Ladies and gentlemen of the jury, you have now heard all the witnesses speak. Everything is on videotape, and during your deliberations you may watch and listen once again to any witness's testimony. In doing so, pay attention not only to what is said, but to how it's said. Does it strike you as truthful? You have a whole lifetime of experience on which you can draw in order to make such a determination.

"In reaching your decision, you must balance what you've heard with your intuition of whether or not, ultimately, you believe you have been told the truth."

Would such a charge to the jury influence the verdict? I have no doubt about it. Do you?

o

VIOLENCE AS NEWS

I saw something on TV the other evening that I wouldn't likely encounter in "real life." A South African black man was forced out of his house and chased by a mob of taunting, stone-throwing youths. Finally they caught up with him and stoned him to death.

"Did that really happen, Daddy, or was that just for TV?" my ten-year-old daughter asked me.

I answered as evasively as I could, while we sipped sodas, that the event we had just witnessed had actually happened. And then she asked me something I couldn't answer.

"Why didn't that man with the camera do something to help?"

Somehow I don't think anything I could have said about "objectivity" or "neutrality" on the part of the electronic media would have been very convincing to a ten-year-old.

Come to think of it, why should it be convincing to those of us who are over ten years of age? Why have we accustomed ourselves to the idea that photographers and video cameramen are merely extensions of the machines that they lug around with them? (People who function as machines are the stuff of science fiction, aren't they?) They're real-life providers of starkly vivid and emotionally depleting images that enter our brain and detonate like a terrorist's bomb.

The human brain, you see, was designed to process only so much raw emotion at one time. If the horrors exceed a certain limit, people start acting strangely in ways that no psychiatrist would have anticipated.

Years ago, "battle fatigue" was a euphemism to describe the emotional breakdown of soldiers who had seen too much: buddies being blown apart by bombs, people taking a round of ammunition full in the face. You know, the kinds of things that the rest of us now routinely watch on the seven o'clock news.

There's a new form of battle fatigue for the 1990s. You don't have to be in the service to get it. You just have to own a television set. And that means we're all potential casualties.

Photography's increasing sophistication radically changed the transmission of information. "Man Jumps to His Death from Brooklyn Bridge" is transformed from an impersonal headline to a horrifying picture taken by a photographer who happened to be nearby of an anguished face looking upward seconds after the leap. Video images increase the dramatic immediacy even further.

Watching a personal tragedy or a natural disaster on the morning news is a qualitatively different experience from merely reading about the tragedy. The video image is processed primarily within the right hemisphere of the brain; it bypasses language, reason, and logic. These terrifying scenes have a psychological impact whose ramifications have not yet been fully understood by TV news executives.

We cannot cope with a sustained assault of elemental emotions like fear, horror, and outrage. If enough horrors are repeatedly depicted with sufficient graphic impact, in a self-protective reflex the brain simply shuts down. Hideous images cease to arouse any emotion except, perhaps, boredom.

In other words, there are only so many pictures of people jumping off the Brooklyn Bridge or being blasted apart by terrorist bombs a person can take before he starts flipping the television dial in a desperate search for a game show. (Is it conceivable that such a possibility may actually prompt TV news executives to mend their ways?)

I'm suggesting that the approach that a picture is more powerful than a thousand words has led to a kind of Gresham's law of the emotions. The stark, the shocking, the bloody, and the horrific numb whatever sensitivities we may still have. Our only choice is to turn off emotionally. The result is a growing insensitivity to the plight of those experiencing hunger, joblessness, pain, and death.

Why do we fail to recognize that it's unhealthy to stir up people's emotions without providing them with some way of expressing their emotions? For years we've recognized the reality of sexual obscenity. Now we must recognize that the depiction of violence is also obscene.

To feed me, along with my dinner, close-ups of bodies of people who have been burned beyond recognition or mutilated by a killer—if that's not obscene and pornographic, what is?

Without knowledge or approval, broadcasters determine when and how we're going to feel moral outrage or disgust or anger. Almost always we can do nothing about these events and situations. Invariably this policy is claiming that these events are happening and therefore people should know about them. Granted. But knowledge of something isn't the same thing as the emotional anxiety seeing it in living color creates.

The visual media—movies, TV, advertising—have so far avoided doing something about the injurious effects on our brains and mental health of being exposed on a daily basis to vividly rendered images of tragedy, horror, and mayhem. These images, thanks to an increasingly sophisticated video technology, can oftentimes be as troubling to our sensibilities as experiencing them in real life.

I would worry about the emotional health of my ten-year-old daughter if she witnessed a terrible fire or a plane crash. And I worry about her peace of mind as she copes with a daily exposure to calamity after calamity on TV.

The pornography of violence is every bit as ugly and brutalizing as sexual pornography—probably more so. Whether you're ten years old or a mature adult, both kinds of pornography are disturbing and antihuman. TV news violence can be dangerous to your mental health.

"I JUST DID IT, I DON'T KNOW WHY"

I am standing between two steel-girded doors. Behind a glass panel to my right a woman guard is giving me a final lookover before activating the automatic door that releases me from the prison.

My situation perfectly mirrors my mental state at the moment: locked between two unyielding and constraining points of view. On the one side is everything that I know about obsessions, jealousy, and murderous rage; opposite are the requirements of the legal system, which after several hundred years has arrived at some very limited ways of dealing with human weaknesses and passions.

One year ago the man that I've just finished interviewing wasn't much different from myself. He was employed, married, the father of three children, a member of clubs, a tennis player. The ordinariness of his life contrasts with his charge: first-degree murder.

Briefly, the story is this: Sixteen years of a reasonably good marriage were punctuated by intermittent episodes of jealousy on the part of Patrick, now forty-two, toward his wife, Connie, thirty-eight at the time of the shooting. Along with a tendency toward jealousy, Patrick periodically erupted into fits of uncontrollable rage marked by feelings of his heart racing, the blood rushing to his head, his head going numb—a sensation, in his own words, "of going completely and irreversibly out of control." On one occasion he became so outraged in response to his wife's failure to account for fifteen minutes of lost time on her way home from work that he destroyed several rooms of the house. He has no memory of this incident. Nor does he recall clearly the final act when the rushing-numb-out-of-control feeling led him to point the gun at his wife and shoot her at point-blank range.

After spending several hours with Patrick, I am reasonably sure that he suffers from a condition known as episodic dyscontrol. According to Russell R. Monroe, the world's expert on the disorder:

> *The dyscontrol act is characterized by feeling, "I just did it, I don't know why." It is an experience of having executed a significant plan without a clear and complete sense of motivation, decision, or sustained wish, so that it does not feel deliberate or fully intended. More often the abrupt precipitous acts are based on primitive emotions of fear, rage or sensuous feelings without concern for the effect on the immediate environment or the long-term consequences to the actor or society and are, therefore, self or socially destructive. These acts are disinhibitions of behavior (in the motor sense) and are often sadistic or bizarre crimes or suicidal attempts.*

What makes episodic dyscontrol different from other forms of "temporary insanity" is that many instances of the disorder are caused by electrical disturbances within the limbic system of the brain—in essence, a rare form of epilepsy. Not all instances of uncontrollable rage (the so-called explosive personality) are based on epilepsy (there is no reason to suppose that Bernhard Goetz, the "subway vigilante" discussed in "The Fiction of the Reasonable Man," suffered from this disorder), but enough cases exist to make my final report a matter of life and death for Patrick. In court I will be asked to give my professional opinion on the question, When Patrick killed his wife (he doesn't deny that he fired the gun that killed her), was he responsible for his actions?

The law in the state where Patrick is imprisoned has this to say about insanity: "The defendant is entitled to acquittal on grounds of insanity if at the time of the commission of the act he either did not know the difference between right and wrong or he was unable to refrain from doing wrong." Certainly there was no doubt Patrick retained his knowledge that to kill his wife was wrong—two psychiatrists have already declared that he is of at least average intelligence and at the moment suffers from no diagnosable psychiatric illness. But was he able to "refrain" from doing wrong— was Patrick capable of shutting off the rage, putting away the gun, talking, reasoning? Or, instead, did he suffer from what the law describes as an "irresistible impulse"?

For centuries such questions were answered by speculations, theorizing, attempts to second-guess the defendant's state of mind. But with the development of new technology a more scientific approach became possible. For instance, the electroencephalogram, or "brain wave test," provided recordings of the brain's spontaneous electrical activity. These recordings, coupled with astute observations of patients, led to the discovery of a distinctive form of epilepsy (complex partial seizures or psychic seizures) emanating from the temporal lobe. During such seizures a storm of abnormal electrical discharges starts somewhere within the limbic system and propagates into the temporal lobe. Because these limbic structures lie deep within the brain, it's not unusual for the standard EEG recordings, employing electrodes attached to the scalp, to be perfectly normal. But if the recordings are made from electrodes implanted deep within the brain, a seizure can often be detected.

To make matters more complicated, even deeply implanted electrodes may sometimes fail to detect a seizure even on occasions when limbic-based epilepsy is strongly suspected. A diagnosis of explosive personality or episodic dyscontrol secondary to limbic discharges, therefore, requires on the part of the neuropsychiatrist a willingness to go beyond the data shown on an EEG. For instance, the doctor must know that people with episodic dyscontrol frequently have a history of head injury in infancy or childhood, encephalitis (inflammation of the brain) early in life, or seizures in infancy; some have a family history of similar temper control problems. In Patrick's history there is head injury, early brain inflammation, and a father with a trigger temper that on one occasion led him to hurl another man out of a second-story window.

But most distinguishing of all in episodic dyscontrol is the nature of the afflicted person's internal experience. Again, Russell Monroe, on irresistible impulses: "The act, itself, might be quite explosive and often aggressive, but is preceded not only by mounting tension but also by a conscious awareness of the impending action, with the realization of the potential disastrous consequences of such action."

From my observations and experience I'm convinced Patrick suffers from episodic dyscontrol. But will an EEG turn up seizure activity? Suppose it's normal? Can I nonetheless convince the jury that Patrick suffers from a disorder leading to an "irresistible impulse"? Further, can I in good faith make such an assertion on Patrick's part? Should I?

The demands of the law and the insights of neuropsychiatry stand in stark contrast in cases like Patrick's. The best that the neuropsychiatrist can do is apply what he knows about the brain and mental illness to the actions of the accused. But because he can never know for certain what went on in the mind of a killer, the neuropsychiatrist must be satisfied with an approximation, a best estimate: "Patrick's early history, his behavior, the observations others have made of him, my own observations—on the basis of all of these, I believe he suffers from an episodic disorder marked by loss of control over his anger. On this basis, I don't believe he was responsible for the killing of his wife."

But the demands of the law are more exacting. First-degree murder requires premeditation, deliberation, and malice. If premeditation or deliberation is not present but malice is, the maximum charge that can be legally sustained will be second-degree murder. If malice is absent but the killer intends to kill his victim, then the crime is voluntary manslaughter. Finally, if the intent to kill is absent, involuntary manslaughter is the charge—assuming there is a reckless disregard for human life. What level of homicide should Patrick be charged with?

More background: several weeks before the killing Patrick purchased a gun. In Patrick's case if premeditation was absent, then what was he going to do with it?

Deliberation, the second requirement, is also difficult to ascertain in the specific instance. During the six months prior to the shooting Patrick was obsessed day and night with thoughts of his failing marriage; his wife's unwillingness to account for every moment of her time; his own crumbling defenses against the rage and jealousy that tore at him. This was not so much deliberation as it was torturous rumination, the daily unending process of thinking thoughts that he didn't want to think. Is sustained anger toward another person sufficient to determine the presence of malice?

In Patrick's case it seems that second-degree murder is the charge that fits the facts best. Obsessive jealousy, sleeplessness, the intake of an unknown quantity of alcohol, and explosive temper—these elements preclude, in my opinion, premeditation and deliberation. This leaves only malice, a state of mind that, in light of the killing, it seems reasonable to conclude Patrick harbored toward his wife.

Put in the simplest terms, a psychiatrist seeks to understand why the accused acted as he did. "To understand all is to forgive all," as one philosopher put it. But, of course, no one—neither I nor anyone else—can put oneself into another person's mind. Even if that could be done, understanding a killer's motives may not be sufficient to absolve the killer from the legal consequences of his actions. That's why another philosopher turned that aphorism I mentioned a moment ago on its head: "To understand all is to forgive nothing."

Consider that Patrick purchased the gun several weeks prior to the killing. Doesn't this prove that he intended to kill, that the murder was premeditated? From the legal point of view that assumption seems to make sense. I say *seems* because close questioning reveals that Patrick actually bought the gun with the purpose of killing himself. At that time he was deeply despondent, recognized that his thought processes were abnormal and, most important, that he couldn't control them. Suicide seemed the best solution. Many a homicide occurs when the inwardly directed anger and guilt in a despondent person is suddenly directed outward. But then Patrick changed his mind. Why not look into things a bit more? he thought. Yet further investigation didn't give him answers. Instead it fed his obsessions. Patrick's mind throughout all this was not a unity but a diversity of warring and contradictory selves. That's why it was possible for Patrick to purchase a gun and still not be clear in his own tortured mind as to the ultimate purpose to which that gun was going to be put. These warring and contradictory selves also made it possible for Patrick to hold that gun and threaten his wife with it while still believing that the gun would not be fired, a life would not be taken.

Such splits within the personality are everyday matters to psychiatrists and neurologists. Indeed, given the splintered, sometimes incoherent conditions of modern life, splits within the self not only are understandable but may, in fact, be the best that any of us could do under the circumstances. Aldous Huxley captured this truth in his essay "Wordsworth in the Tropics":

> The only satisfactory way of existing in the modern, highly specialized world is to live with two personalities. A Dr. Jekyll that does the metaphysical and scientific thinking, that transacts business in the city, adds up figures, designs machines, and so forth. And a natural, spontaneous Mr. Hyde to do the physical instinctive living in the intervals of work. The two personalities should lead their unconnected lives apart, without poaching on one another's preserves or inquiring too closely into one another's activities. Only by living discretely and inconsistently can we preserve both the man and the citizen, both the intellectual and the spontaneous animal being, alive within us. The solution may not be satisfactory; but it is, I believe now (though once I thought differently), the best that, under modern circumstances, can be devised.

But what is to be done with Mr. Hyde when Dr. Jekyll commits a murder? I ask myself as the inner steel-girded doors finally open and I step out of the prison. As I walk toward the chain-link fence, I can see in my mind's eye the jury that several months from now Patrick and I will be facing together. How convincing I will be on his behalf may mean for Patrick the difference between life and death, freedom and perpetual confinement.

o

EASY
IN THE ISLANDS

It lies there in my hands, curled up into a cold, furry ball. With an effort I can open it up, separating the face and head from the tail and rump. But as soon as I cease applying force, the squirrel curls back into the ball: what else could this be but rigor mortis, the rigidity of death?

"But that squirrel is not dead at all," says biologist Brian Barnes. Taking the creature from my hands, he forcefully straightens its body with a motion that reminds me of opening a blade in a Swiss army knife.

After the maneuver is repeated a few times (the small animal curling back up into a cold, furry ball; Barnes straightening it out again), the animal makes its first movements: tiny motions of its feet, some shaking of its head.

The animal in question is a hibernating arctic squirrel, a member of a class officially known as *Spermophilus parryii*. The place is a laboratory at the Institute of Arctic Biology, University of Alaska, Fairbanks. The time is late afternoon, about three hours before my lecture at the university on the subject of the human brain.

In order to restore the ground squirrel to "life," it is necessary only to place it in a heated environment, like this laboratory. If one is sufficiently patient, the same thing will happen outdoors sometime between September and April or May. At that time the animal becomes "alive," moves, eats, scurries around, and acts positively squirrel-like.

My interest in the ground squirrel dates from an observation made more than fifty years ago by a German scientist. He made the point that many animals survive in harsh environments by making behavioral and physical adaptations similar to those made by manic and depressed patients. Like the hibernating arctic squirrel, such patients may at different times eat heavily or lightly; gain or lose weight; become active or lethargic; undergo great variations in their sleep requirements, their interest in sex, and their interaction with the world around them.

"In the winter just about everybody up here sleeps in, particularly over the weekend," a scientist mentioned to me earlier over lunch in Fairbanks. "The almost total darkness does something to you. No matter how many things you have to do, no matter how personally ambitious you may be about your particular project— that darkness and cold presents an insurmountable barrier to your getting out of bed."

That same scientist went on to describe in himself and his friends (none of them particularly depressed or elated) the same trends exhibited to a more profound degree by some of the patients I have treated over the years for depression: increased appetite, particularly for carbohydrates; weight gain; loss of energy; the need for more sleep.

"With the coming of spring, most of us make up for all that torpor," he said. "It is not unusual for people to go on only four hours of sleep a night over the entire summer. We even have a softball game up here that doesn't get started until eleven-thirty or twelve o'clock at night."

Variations in mood and activity in response to the seasons were first described by no less a figure than Hippocrates, the Father of Medicine. "It is chiefly the changes of the seasons which produce diseases, and in the seasons the great changes are from cold or heat." By the fourth century A.D. the pattern was identified. "Melancholy occurs in autumn, whereas mania in summer," wrote Posidonius, a Stoic philosopher (I can't help wondering what a Stoic would have made of the arctic).

Additional observations over the centuries revealed that seasonal mood changes conform to two seasonal patterns rather than to one: recurrent winter depression (by far the most common) and recurrent summer depression. Hippocrates observed in an aside that "of constitutions, some are well or ill adapted to summer, others are well or ill adapted to winter."

Included among summer depressives are those who complain about the heat and humidity of summer days and suffer from lack of energy. The poet John Milton, who suffered from summer depression, told an acquaintance that "his vein never happily flowed but from the autumnal equinoctial to the vernal, and that whatever he attempted [in summer] was never to his satisfaction . . . so that all the years he was about this poem [*Paradise Lost*] he may be said to have spent but half his time therein."

Paradise Lost is a "winter" book meant to be read by the fireside, to the rhythms of crackling logs, snow on frozen windowpanes. Indeed, it is hard to imagine its being written or even read under the hot, humid, hazy conditions of a typical summer day. So, too, with any work by Kierkegaard, Dostoevsky, or Freud—definitely winter people. But not so with Cervantes, Gabriel García Márquez, Joseph Conrad—these writers exert their greatest appeal during the longish days of summer.

Clearly creativity doesn't exist in a vacuum: Cervantes would have done poorly in Copenhagen; somehow one can't imagine Kierkegaard writing *A Sickness unto Death* while sitting in a garden in Madrid. Like it or not, seasonal and environmental influences exert powerful effects on our personalities, moods, proclivities.

Nor is this influence limited to the strikingly creative. A 1988 survey revealed that 5 percent of the population in Montgomery County, Maryland, a Washington, D.C., suburb, experienced seasonal depressions as severe as patients enrolled in a seasonal depression clinic. The tricky point, it seems, is deciding whether one's low spirits occur primarily in the summer or in the winter.

Once that is decided upon, the treatment is fairly straightforward. As one of the earliest examples on record the psychiatrist Jean Esquirol advised in 1845 that one of his patients suffering from winter depression "be in Italy before the close of October, from whence you must not return until the month of May." Esquirol was firmly convinced of the value of this treatment method of "climatotherapy"; it would endear him to travel agents forever after.

In my own case, I can still recall the intensity of my feelings the first time I stepped off an airplane on a beautiful sunny January afternoon in the Caribbean. Three hours earlier I had precipitously fled New York's rain, cold, and loneliness in an effort to revive my seriously lagging spirits. As I stepped from the plane and felt the sun on my face, I started to cry—probably the only "tears of joy" that I have ever shed in my life. At that time—the late sixties— very little was known about seasonal depression, and I doubt that any of my fellow passengers understood what I was feeling at the moment. Instinctively, though, I knew that it was the *light* that was making me so happy.

This idea of light and darkness as influences on one's mood can be traced back many centuries. Greek and Roman doctors thought of depression as a kind of internal darkness. In the second century the physician Galen wrote that "the color of the black humor induces fear when its darkness throws a shadow over the area of thought. . . ."

If darkness is the disease, then light must be the cure. This simplistic concept was applied 2000 years before my first of many annual January trips to the Caribbean. "Lethargics are to be laid in the light and exposed to the rays of the sun (for the disease is gloom)," wrote the physician Aretaus in the second century.

But it wasn't until 1946 that the description of phototherapy— exposure of the depressed person to bright light—first appeared in a medical journal. Since then, numerous experimental trials— most of them conducted at the National Institute of Mental Health by Thomas A. Wehr and Norman E. Rosenthal—have attested to the beneficial influence of bright light on winter depression, or

SAD (seasonal affective disorder), as it's now called. Depending on time, circumstances, and one's financial situation, the depressed person can sit before one of the artificial "light boxes" that have become so popular, or flee to the Caribbean.

In either case what is needed is the same experience that made me cry tears of joy: bright light entering the eye, traveling along the optic nerve to the suprachiasmatic nucleus of the hypothalamus, and from there to the pineal—the solitary midline structure that Descartes considered the seat of the soul.

At the pineal light inhibits the regular nocturnal secretion of melatonin. Thus a bright light directed into the eyes induces a response within the brain similar to what happens in the summer: a shortening of the duration of melatonin secretion.

The influence of light and seasonality on moods isn't a concept that does a lot for one's sense of autonomy. In our heart of hearts most of us like to think that we are always in control of our feelings. (Of course, *others* may be dominated by sunlight, temperature, and who knows what other environmental variables, "but not *me*," most of us proclaim, often with an intense display of feeling.) In my own case, though, I gladly accept my need for sun and light. Without that yearly trip to the Caribbean I am moody, cranky, "impossible to live with" (my wife's words).

I am thinking of all of these things as I take into my hands the cold and rigid Alaskan ground squirrel. I can readily identify with that creature's withdrawal, taciturnity, and forced immobility. But in contrast to the ground squirrel, we can, on the basis of our awareness of the seasons' effects on our moods, choose to move toward more accommodating realms.

No . . . it is not likely that I will think of returning to Fairbanks when I plan next year's winter vacation. Instead of a mug of steaming tea I will order a rum punch; instead of pondering the depths of the permafrost table, I'll be happily applying sun protection ointment while sitting somewhere on a secluded beach in the Caribbean.

My motto is that of the elderly native I met last winter in Saint

Kitts. While standing just at the waterline and smiling into the sunlight, he looked up at me and asked, "Mon . . . isn't it easier in the Islands?"

"Right, mon," I answered, smiling at him, enjoying the warmth of the sun as it bathed my face, my body, my very soul in light.

DECADE
OF THE BRAIN

In a July 25, 1989, Oval Office ceremony President Bush signed into law the only bill in history dedicated to a human organ. H.J. Res. 174 proclaims the years 1990 to 2000 the Decade of the Brain.

Meanwhile, across town and at about the same time, Congress, not to be preempted, was working with the Advisory Panel on the Neurosciences, established one year earlier. At congressional request this panel of experts in fields ranging from psychiatry to ethics to collective bargaining was holding regular meetings on Capitol Hill under the auspices of the Office of Technology Assessment. The purpose of the panel? To advise Congress about advances in the brain sciences likely to make the greatest impact upon life in the twenty-first century.

Why this sudden government interest in things neurological?

For one thing, it has not escaped politicians of every persuasion that brain science is in striking distance of favorably affecting, if not necessarily curing, a smorgasbord of illnesses afflicting Americans from cradle to grave. Alzheimer's disease in the elderly; brain injuries and developmental difficulties in infants and children; multiple sclerosis in young adults; schizophrenia and manic-depression across the life span—these are only some of the conditions where important breakthroughs are expected.

195

Important factors contributing to this new optimism about the brain include these:

• Recent advances in imaging techniques. These started in the 1970s with CAT scans, which represented a quantum leap in visualization. Thanks to CAT scans, radiologists and doctors caring for patients were able for the first time to study computer-generated and computer-assisted pictures of structures too deep within the brain to be seen by traditional X rays. With the arrival of MRI scans, employing powerful magnets instead of radiation, the resolving power of visual imaging techniques was vastly increased (down to the millimeter level). But both CAT and MRI scans provide, for the most part, only static images. It wasn't until the early 1980s that the dynamic functioning brain was revealed in all of its wonder by means of PET scans. These multicolored pictures displayed ongoing metabolism within brain areas active under specific conditions, like listening to music, reading, and talking. In one famous experiment, a PET scan showed the brain concentrating intently on moving the subject's hand but without actually doing so.

• Computer-assisted enhancements of the information provided by EEGs. Thanks to these instruments, which carry names like BEAM (brain electrical activity map), neuroscientists can watch video displays of the electrical "storm" within the brain during epileptic seizures. Researchers are already noting distinctive brain wave patterns in some people with dyslexia and other learning problems.

• Advances in our understanding of the chemistry of the brain— the most powerful contributors to the emerging enthusiasm for the neurological sciences. Neuroscientists now know that information is processed within the brain via perhaps as many as 150 brain messengers, including such chemical message-bearing substances as neurotransmitters, peptides, and small molecular compounds like the same amino acids that make up our diet. Moreover, disturbances in these transmitter substances can result in specific neurological and psychiatric diseases—for example, Parkinson's, where the neurotransmitter dopamine is deficient. The most recent and exciting finding is that some forms of depression may be largely the result of an abnormality of a single neurotransmitter. For instance, the most popular antidepressant in history, Prozac, works by influencing the levels of serotonin within the brain.

On the basis of this three-pronged, technologically driven attack on the brain, neuroscientists anticipate that brain research holds great promise, as well as some peril, during the Decade of the Brain. At the moment the congressional advisory group is grappling with the scientific, social, ethical, and political implications of the following:

Neurotoxicology (the study of substances capable of poisoning the brain and nervous system). Because of its structural and chemical complexity, the brain is particularly at risk from toxic agents. Along with environmental pollutants like carbon monoxide, lead, and mercury, commonly encountered neurotoxic agents include food additives, drugs, and industrial and occupational chemicals. Indeed, one would have to lead a hermit's life to shield oneself from all agents in the environment with the potential for harming the brain. So far, not much is known about the extent of the damage some of these agents can bring about within the brain, but neuroscientists are hopeful that measures may be taken that will prevent future brain damage.

Neural transplants and nerve regeneration. Included here are efforts to treat brain diseases by replacing injured brain parts with tissue taken from other parts of the body, such as the adrenal gland, or from the brains of aborted fetuses. In either case the aim is to replace needed chemicals lost as a result of disease.

A considerable degree of controversy can be expected as to whether the prochoice position should be extended to include a woman's right to contribute to brain research by selling at a profit the remains of the child she has chosen not to carry to term. This moral dilemma is just one of the reasons the advisory panel includes ethicists as well as neuroscientists.

So far, between three hundred and four hundred persons with

Parkinson's disease have received neural grafts. Whether this approach will be successful with other neurological illnesses remains uncertain. Parkinson's disease, in contrast to most other target diseases, involves the grafting of only a small amount of neural tissue to a very specific site within the brain. Also, only one neurotransmitter, dopamine, needs replacement.

Biological rhythms and shift work. Today one out of five workers in the United States do not work a nine-to-five shift. Despite this high percentage of nontraditional work hours, very little information exists regarding potential behavioral and neurological harm. The information that does exist indicates that irregular shift work exacts a high toll in terms of lowered job performance ratings, decreased worker satisfaction, more sick days, and higher rates of psychological disturbance and substance abuse.

The biological basis for mental illness. As a result of biochemical research on tranquilizers and antidepressant drugs, scientists have learned that the major forms of mental illness (schizophrenia, manic depression) are associated with and perhaps even caused by chemical disturbances within the brain. The branch of psychiatry representing this view of mental illness, variously described as biological psychiatry or neuropsychiatry, is at the moment the most promising and exciting avenue of research within the field. Among the questions addressed by the congressional panel are these: Will all forms of emotional illness and disturbance turn out to be ultimately biological in origin? Should treatment approaches be directed primarily to the biological dimension, or should social and psychological factors continue to be given some measure of credibility via psychotherapy and counseling?

Along with this interest in the operation of the brain as a whole, scientists are excited about what can be learned about the brain from the study of any one of the brain's three hundred billion or so individual neurons. Just as an investigator can learn a great deal about the workings of a large city by interviewing one of its better-informed inhabitants, so neuroscientists are betting that the detailed investigation of processes on the cellular level may yield important facts about such things as memory. The work of Eric Kandel on the retention powers of the lowly sea slug (a creature with neurons numbering in the hundreds of thousands rather than millions) hints at the possibility that nature may, in the interest of efficiency, have designed a memory-encoding mechanism at the cellular level and then retained it for creatures, like ourselves, with vastly more complicated nervous systems.

Despite not being comparable to brains, computers will continue to provide essential assistance in brain research. Computer graphics are already making possible subtle alterations in the chemical structure of compounds. Within the past two years neuroscientists have come up with the discovery of the receptor in the brain for marijuana. They have even succeeded in cloning the gene for its receptor. Next on the horizon will be computer-aided alterations of the marijuana molecule so as to allow the development of a family compound that retains marijuana's beneficial effects (it cuts back on the nausea that some cancer patients experience during their chemotherapy) while doing away with the substance's central effects (few cancer patients wish to live the rest of their lives "stoned").

Other attempts to alter the brain on the molecular level involve innovative partnerships between brain scientists and molecular geneticists. Huntington's disease and certain forms of depression already have been traced to distinct locations on human chromosomes. An important goal of the human gene project is correlating specific brain and behavioral disorders with specific genetic locations. Once this is done, the chromosomes can be identified.

When scientists locate the chromosome abnormality associated with a particular brain disease, they hope to be in a position to suggest some forms of treatment. These may include inserting genetic material produced in other organisms (cloning), altering the patient's genetic code, or introducing the part of the chromosome that is deficient, defective, or, in some cases, missing altogether.

Another method of gene therapy might involve intercepting the "message" as it passes from genes to proteins via messenger RNA.

This may be a particularly desirable treatment approach because altering messenger RNA rather than the defective gene itself is likely to be less technically demanding. For one thing, it requires altering not the actual gene but only the garbled message that results when the abnormal gene communicates its message to RNA for transmission into the body of the nerve cell. "Dealing with the middleman" may also be desirable because any specific site on a chromosome may carry out *several* functions, only one of which may be abnormal.

Events within the neuron are also turning out to be important when it comes to predicting the consequences of a neurotransmitter's interacting with its receptor. Neuroscientists have discovered that this is far more complicated and interactive than anyone believed only a few years ago. Rather than a simple one-to-one relationship of transmitter to receptor, which then results in a single response, the neurotransmitter may activate its receptor to release a "second messenger," which then, like a pinball, activates many other reactions. The process is called a "cascade reaction," and the brain thrives on it. Recently "third messengers" have been turning up, producing a larger number of possible combinations of chemical reactions between brain chemicals and their receptors than could be handled by even the most powerful computer presently imaginable.

As the result of the new molecular approach to the brain, neuroscientists no longer believe that many neurological or psychiatric diseases will turn out to be caused by disturbances in single neurotransmitters. It is likely that most brain diseases will turn out to involve several chemicals and components of the brain. Therefore, more than simple replacement therapy, like in Parkinson's disease, will be needed. Even Parkinson's, once considered the paramount example of a disease resulting from a comparatively simple chemical defect (a decrease in dopamine) is now recognized as much more complicated and involving other neurotransmitters as well. As a result of this very recent insight, sufferers from Parkinson's disease are now treated with drugs that effect changes in one form of an important brain enzyme, monoamine oxidase, which was formerly considered important in depression.

Given these varied and far-ranging avenues of research on the human brain planned over the next ten years, it seems reasonable to hope that the Decade of the Brain will live up to its promise. And if it does, imagine the benefits that could result if we could learn, say, what happens within the brain when we feel angry, or sad, or—best of all—happily contented with our lives.

o

BIBLIOGRAPHY

Changeux, Jean-Pierre. *Neuronal Man* (New York: Pantheon Books, 1985).

Granit, Ragnar. *The Purposive Brain* (Cambridge, Mass.: The MIT Press, 1977).

Gregory, Richard. *The Oxford Companion to the Mind* (New York: Oxford University Press, 1987).

Restak, Richard M. *The Brain: The Last Frontier* (New York: Doubleday, 1979; available in paperback from Warner Books).

———. *The Brain* (New York: Bantam, 1984; available in paperback from Bantam).

———. *The Infant Mind* (New York: Doubleday, 1986).

———. *The Mind* (New York: Bantam, 1988).

Spillane, John D. *The Doctrine of the Nerves: Chapters in the History of Neurology* (New York: Oxford University Press, 1981).

INDEX